Documentation in a SNAP

For Activity Programs
Fourth Edition

with MDS 3.0

Ann G Uniack, RHIA

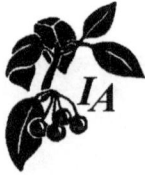

Idyll Arbor, Inc.

39129 264th Ave SE, Enumclaw, WA 98022 (360) 825-7797

This publication is based on guidelines published by the Centers for Medicare and Medicaid Services (CMS). State and local regulations and laws may vary. The examples in this book are meant as guidelines only. The implementation is the responsibility of the nursing facility.

All names, histories, and conditions in the publication are fictitious. Any similarity to persons living or dead is purely coincidental.

Idyll Arbor Editor: Thomas M. Blaschko

S N A P is the trademark of S.N.A.P., Inc.
Documentation is a SNAP is the trademark of a series of publications written by Ann G. Uniack.

ISBN: 9781882883936

Printed in the United States of America

Library of Congress Cataloging-in-Publication Data

Uniack, Ann G.
  Documentation in a SNAP for activity programs with MDS 3.0 / Ann G. Uniack. -- 4th ed.
      p. ; cm.
  Includes index.
  ISBN 978-1-882883-93-6
  I. Skilled Nursing Assessment Programs. II. Title.
  [DNLM: 1. Nursing Assessment--methods. 2. Documentation--methods. 3. Long-Term Care--organization & administration. 4. Medical Records. 5. Quality Assurance, Health Care--methods. 6. Skilled Nursing Facilities--organization & administration. WY 100.4]

  651.5'04261--dc23

                                                                    2011049139

Write it concise

Never write it twice

Contents

INTRODUCTION

Charting is never a SNAP! And it is often a low priority. An activity professional's first interest is working with people. And rightly so.

Energy is directed toward improving the quality of life for residents in the nursing facility. Each resident has special needs. Success is measured by positive outcomes of care. To achieve positive outcomes, the interdisciplinary team must coordinate a plan of care that is right for each resident.

The purpose of this book is to create a system of documentation that supports the delivery of resident care. The clinical record may be either handwritten or electronic. But its purpose is to provide the activity professional with information to:

- assess each resident's needs,
- develop a plan of care,
- establish goals to be achieved and outcomes expected,
- document interventions, and
- evaluate the success or need for revision of the care plan.

Throughout this book there are references specific to the activity program in a nursing facility. Included within the chapters are references that apply to activity programs from federal regulations with interpretive guidelines and from the Resident Assessment Instrument (RAI) Version 3.0 Manual published by the Centers for Medicare and Medicaid Services (CMS). (These references are boxed in bold or italic type.) One can't play the game without knowing the rules.

Information is the key to meeting residents' needs. Health professionals turn to the clinical record for that information. Whether paper based or computerized, in order for the clinical record to be useful, accurate, and easy to find, documentation must be available for staff to make decisions for resident care.

In other words, DOCUMENTATION must be a SNAP!

1. CLINICAL RECORD GUIDELINES

KEY POINTS AND SUMMARY OF CHAPTER

The clinical record whether written by hand or computer is a legal document that is evidence of resident care.

Documentation in the clinical record must follow the rules for recording in a legal document.

All resident information is organized and maintained in the clinical record to allow easy access for all health care providers.

Resident health information must be protected from loss, tampering, or unauthorized access.

A. Legal Document

The clinical record is a business record. Records made in the regular course of business and at the time an event occurred are legal documents. Documentation in the clinical record is completed by members of the interdisciplinary team who have knowledge of the acts, events, conditions, opinions, or diagnoses concerning the resident. The clinical record is the evidence of the care that was given.

There are four requirements that must be met for the clinical record to be considered as evidence by a Court of Law.

- The record was documented in the normal course of business.
- The record was written at or near the time care was given.
- A person with knowledge of the resident's care completed the documentation in the record.
- The record was stored in a safe and secure manner to prevent loss, tampering, or unauthorized use.

When a health care professional completes clinical record documentation in a timely manner, that information is presumed to be true. A Court of Law considers the clinical record as the proof of work performed. It is often said, *If it was not documented, it was not done.*

A health care professional may sign a time sheet or punch a time clock to prove that he or she was present at work. But what is the proof that the person provided care to any residents? The proof is the documentation in the clinical record, such as assessments, progress notes, attendance records, and flow sheets of one-to-one visits. If documentation is not complete, there is no proof that a person has done his or her job. When records are not completed on time, the information can become suspect. An accurate health record is the best proof of care.

B. Rules for Documentation

Because the clinical record is a legal document that is evidence of care, it is maintained according to written, approved facility procedures, as well as state and federal regulations. Rules for recording in legal documents must be followed. If the rules for recording are not followed, the clinical record will not be considered accurate or true.

> For example, consider documents that are handled in one's daily life. Credit card receipts and personal checks are legal documents. The person in possession of those documents can expect to be paid or to be obligated to pay the amount that is stated on the paper. These documents are business records completed in the regular course of business according to rules for recording on legal documents.

Now think about the clinical record. The clinical record is a legal document. It is proof that care was provided to the resident. It is evidence of the kind and quality of care given to a resident. The same principles that are used to write a check or complete a credit card transaction apply to the clinical record. Carefully follow the rules for recording to make sure that your documentation is legal.

1. Legible

The entries in the clinical record must be clearly written so other health care professionals can understand the entry. Often handwritten notes are made hastily and errors occur, which then are not corrected in a legible manner. Or staff may use abbreviations that are not approved as shorthand, limiting another reader's understanding. Allow enough time to make thoughtful and clearly written entries.

Some factors that may hinder legibility and put resident care at risk are

- Poor handwriting,
- Use of unauthorized abbreviations,
- Felt tip pens,
- Improper corrections of errors, or
- Low toner or ink in computer printer cartridge.

Easy access to documentation allows the interdisciplinary team to get the information they need to give care. Documentation that is clearly written and legible allows staff to give the best care.

2. Ink, Typewritten, Printed by Computer

All entries in the clinical record should be original documents and be written in permanent ink, typewritten, or printed by a computer. It is best to use a medium point blue or black ballpoint pen. Colored ink, especially in fine point pens, can be difficult to read or photocopy. Some felt tip pens are not permanent and are erasable. In addition, entries made by felt tip pens may be illegible or may bleed through the paper, making documentation on the reverse side of the page impossible to read.

Pencil may not be used. Remember the example of writing a personal check. It would be unthinkable for a person to write a check in pencil. An erasure would easily change the amount of money specified. The same holds true for documentation of resident care.

3. Dated

Each entry in the clinical record is dated. It is both unethical and illegal to pre-date or post-date an entry. Entries in the clinical record are identified with the date and time they are made. Documentation should be completed as soon as possible after an event or observation occurs.

Always include the year when writing dates. A complete date including the year is essential to identify the time frame of each entry throughout the entire record. Many residents stay longer than one year and some for a number of years. Complete dates and even times may be needed to document a situation accurately.

Using only month and year for quarterly notes is not recommended. The resident's condition at the beginning of a month may be significantly different from the condition thirty days later. For example, a resident may suddenly have a change of condition during the month. If the entry did not include the day of the month, it might appear that the activity professional was unaware of the change in condition.

4. Signature with Full Name and Title

Every entry in the clinical record must be validated with a signature, either handwritten or electronic. Again, consider the example of writing a personal check. If the check does not have a signature, the bank will not cash the check. If a credit card receipt does not have a signature, the amount due may not be honored.

The complete name and professional title of the person making the entry authenticates that entry. Health care professionals must always write and sign their own entries. Never make an entry or sign an entry for someone else.

An electronic signature is created on a computer by entering a unique code or password that verifies the identity of the person who completed the documentation. The signature line printed by the computer usually states "Electronically signed by Mary Smith, Activity Director on (date and time)." This is not the same as the computer printing a person's name on a signature line without any authentication.

Accessing a computer program with a password does not mean that there is an electronic signature. Each documentation entry must be specifically authenticated to be an electronic signature. The CMS's RAI Version 3.0 User's Manual states that nursing homes may use electronic signatures for clinical record documentation, including the

MDS, when permitted to do so by state and local law and when authorized by the long-term care facility's policy.

Information may be transcribed into the clinical record from a source completed by another health care professional. When doing so, identify the name and title of the person transcribing the information, and the name and title of the person who originally wrote the information.

> For example, *Transcribed by Mary Jones, Activity Director, from Transfer Record (date) signed by Susan Smith, RN.*

Data entry by clerical staff into computer systems from handwritten worksheets is not considered transcription. The health care professional that completed the worksheet must review the computer printout and authenticate the information as correct with a complete signature.

> For example, Minimum Data Set (MDS) assessment information may be entered from a handwritten document into the computer by medical record staff. The Activity Professional who completed the information for Section F of the MDS will need to sign the certification statement on the MDS to verify that data in Section F are accurate.

5. Initials

Federal regulations state that full signatures and titles are required on the Minimum Data Set (MDS) assessment. Initials may be used on flow sheets if the signature of the health care professional is also recorded somewhere on that same flow sheet.

Initials of the health care professional's name should not be used to authenticate narrative notes or assessments. Initials can be difficult to decipher and may cause problems with identifying the person who actually made an entry.

6. Completing Forms

When completing forms or checklists, all questions and fields need to be answered. If the item is not applicable, mark the area as n/a. Fields or questions left blank may lead to confusion. A reviewer does not know if the information was omitted or was not applicable (N/A).

When completing Section F of the MDS, follow the CMS's RAI Version 3.0 Manual instructions on using any dashes, skips, or not applicable. The computer program will identify any MDS entries that do not follow the rules.

7. Corrections

When there is an error in documentation, make a legal correction. Do not attempt to erase, write-over, block out, or use whiteout. Strict rules apply to correcting clinical records. Improper corrections will invalidate the record for legal purposes. When records are unclear, they can affect resident care and become a liability.

For example, a personal check or credit card receipt with whiteout would not be valid. Likewise, a clinical record that has not been corrected properly would no longer be evidence of care.

To make a legal correction, follow these steps:

- Draw a single line through each word, phrase, or line of the written material to be corrected. Make sure that the original information remains legible. Do not obliterate the information to be corrected.
- State that the information was a "Correction," then write the date and initial the documentation to be corrected.
- Next record the correct information. The person making the correction then signs the entry with complete name and professional title.

If an entire page is in error and must be recopied, the original may not be discarded. The original page is marked as recopied, signed and dated by the person doing the transcription and filed with the corrected copy. The original entry made at the time the event occurred, along with the signature of the professional authenticating the notes, must always be available with the recopied material.

Computer entries to the clinical record may be corrected until the assessment or notes are completed, authenticated by electronic signature, and locked. Once a computer entry is finalized, it can no longer be changed. Follow regulations and facility procedures for making corrections and addenda to computerized records. Software programs will identify how to add corrections and addenda to the record without deleting the original documentation.

8. Omissions in Documentation

At times it will be necessary to make an entry that is out of sequence or provide additional documentation to supplement or clarify entries previously written. These types of entries in the clinical record are identified as Late Entry, Addendum, or Clarification.

Such entries may be used for assessments, orders, or narrative notes:

- Late Entry is documentation made when a pertinent or required entry was missed or not written in a timely manner. Late entries are made when documentation was not completed during the time period required, such as a late quarterly progress note.
- Addendum is used to provide additional information that was not included in the original chart entry. For example, information may be added to the chart about reasons that were later identified regarding why a resident did not receive a treatment or a refusal of treatment.
- Clarification is written to add information to an original entry to avoid misinterpretation. Most often, clarifications are made to physician orders. For example, a physician may write an order that a resident may have a leave of absence for a weekend. The clarification may be necessary to indicate that the leave of absence is for the resident's birthday weekend at a daughter's home.

The following steps are used to document out of sequence entries:

- Identify the type of entry (Late Entry, Addendum, or Clarification) with current date and time.
- Refer to the date and type of documentation (Assessment, Orders, Progress Note) that will be amended.
- Complete the additional information and sign with name and title.

Examples:

(Current Date) Late entry for quarterly progress note
(Due date that was missed)

(Current Date) Addendum to Initial Assessment
(Date of initial assessment)

(Current Date) Clarification to Physician Order
(Date of physician order)

Clinical documentation should always be done in a timely manner. Do not falsify the record by pre-dating or post-dating an entry.

Take care to make sure that chart entries are timely, complete, and accurate. Frequent entries identified as Late Entry may raise questions about the accuracy of all the information contained in a clinical record.

9. Chronological Order

The progress notes in the chart must be maintained in chronological order. Health professionals expect to find information in predictable places in the clinical record. If reports are out of order, the information may not be found when needed. Incomplete information may lead to decisions that are not in the best interests of the resident.

Entries are recorded consecutively in the clinical record. Do not leave spaces or skip lines to allow someone else to document. When it is necessary to leave a blank section at the bottom of the progress notes and begin a new sheet of paper, line out that section of the progress note that is being left blank. The purpose of lining out the blank lines is to prevent someone from writing in the blank space. This is a protection for record integrity and will help keep the chart in chronological order.

10. Continued Notes to Next Page

When a progress note is continued onto another page, write continued at the end of the page. This will show that the entry is completed on the next page. On the new page, indicate the date again, write continued, and record the remainder of the note. Conclude the documentation with a full signature.

By writing on both sheets that there is continued information on another page, those reviewing the notes are alerted that additional details of care are recorded elsewhere. If continuations are not clearly identified, decisions could be made with incomplete information, increasing the risk of errors in treatment.

Guidelines for maintaining a legal document need to be followed to assure the integrity of the clinical record. Records need to be stored to prevent loss of pages from the record and to prevent any damage or destruction from the elements. These guidelines apply to both paper and computerized records.

To be useful, the clinical record must be systematically organized. Reports must be clearly identified with resident's name. Care should be taken to avoid misfiling reports. The purpose of the clinical record is to provide accurate, concise, comprehensive health information about the resident.

More and more nursing homes are maintaining clinically records electronically on computers. Federal regulations allow the clinical records, including the MDS, to be maintained on computers. The maintenance of parts of the clinical record electronically does not require that the entire record must be computerized. In the case that some records are maintained in the computer and some in paper form, the system is known as a hybrid record. The facility must have policies and procedures for how the chart will be maintained.

1. Unit Record

All resident health information must be centralized in the clinical record. Missing or late documentation may lead to unintentional errors by others who depend on the record for information. The health care professional must know all the facts to make decisions. Quality care is not possible if information is not timely, incomplete, or inaccurate.

> For example, if the activity professional is not informed that a resident is diabetic, snacks may be offered during a food-related activity that would not be appropriate for that resident. Although the activity professional has followed all regulations and standards of performance, a poor outcome may result for the resident. A diabetic resident may not be able to tolerate a snack that is too high in sugar or carbohydrates and should be provided with an alternate suitable snack.

Complete and accurate information is the key to assuring quality care. Social Service assessments, care plans, and progress notes must be completed on time. Positive outcomes can only be achieved if all health care professionals are working together, making decisions on reliable information. The clinical record is the source of resident health information for all members of the interdisciplinary team.

2. Clinical Record Organization

The current record is usually maintained in a binder with section tabs for the various health care disciplines. Activity program documentation will have its own tab divider. Be careful that all documentation is filed behind the correct divider. Misfiled reports can cause problems when health care professionals are not able to find the information needed.

If a resident stays for a long time and the chart becomes bulky, sections of the record may be thinned by medical record personnel. Such thinned records are usually maintained near the nursing station or in the medical record department. Initial activity assessments should remain in the chart as baseline documentation. However, progress notes, monitoring tools, and other flow sheets may be thinned out according to facility policy, such as after fifteen months or two years.

3. Report Identification

Every page in the clinical record or computerized record screen must identify the resident by name, record number, and room location in the facility. This identification should be on both sides of every page that is handwritten or computer printed.

Resident identification information can be hand-written in ink, typewritten, printed by computer, stamped using an addressograph machine, or affixed by a label.

4. Photocopies

The clinical record should contain original documents of reports completed by facility staff. Photocopied reports from other hospitals, laboratories, or outside providers may be included as part of the record.

Copies used as part of the clinical record must be permanent copies, such as from a photocopy or plain paper fax machine. Carbon copies, NCR (no carbon required), or thermal fax copies may fade or become illegible over time. Use these reports only on a temporary basis. If necessary, photocopy the temporary reports received on such paper. Retain the permanent photocopy in the clinical record. Discard the temporary fax copy in a confidential manner.

The availability of health information to others providing care for the resident is important to assure continuity and proper care. The clinical record may be duplicated so health information can be made available to other hospitals or health care providers. However, the original report always stays in the facility clinical record.

The clinical record must be written in a manner so that a legible photocopy or fax can be made. Intensely colored paper may not make a legible photocopy. Colored ink may be used, if the facility's photocopy equipment can clearly reproduce the record.

5. Facsimile (FAX) Copies

Fax copies are acceptable in the clinical record. A signature on the fax copy is valid according to federal laws. The original author does not have to countersign the fax copy when later visiting the facility. The original copy may be maintained at the originator's office to be produced upon request. Or the original may be sent to the nursing facility to be included in the clinical record and the fax copy may be discarded in a confidential manner.

D. Abbreviations

An approved abbreviation list should be maintained at the facility. This list is reviewed periodically to assure that the abbreviations used have been approved. A list of generally accepted abbreviations is shown in the box below.

COMMONLY USED ABBREVIATIONS

AD	Activity Director	neg	negative
ADL	activities of daily living	NF	nursing facility
AKA	above the knee amputation	NKA	no known allergies
AM	morning (before noon)	noc	night
A&O	alert and oriented	NPO	nothing by mouth
BKA	below the knee amputation	NWB	non-weight bearing
CAA	Care Area Assessment	OOB	out of bed
c/o	complaint of	PM	afternoon/evening
cont	continued	prn	as needed
DOB	date of birth	PTA	prior to admission
Dx	diagnosis	RAI	Resident Assessment Instrument
ETOH	ethanol (alcohol)	ROM	range of motion
Fx	fracture	SNF	skilled nursing facility
HOH	hard of hearing	STAT	immediately
Hx	history of	TPR	temperature, pulse, & respiration
IDT	interdisciplinary team	TTWB	touch toe weight bearing
LOA	leave of absence	Tx	treatment
LN	licensed nurse	w/c	wheelchair
MD	medical doctor, physician	WNL	within normal limits
MDS	Minimum Data Set	wt	weight

Health care professionals who use abbreviations should ask for approval of all abbreviations that they intend to use. Approval is obtained from the committee that reviews resident care policies or quality assessment and assurance.

Use only facility-approved abbreviations. Studies have shown that some abbreviations contribute to medical errors. The Joint Commission on Accreditation of Hospitals and Organizations has identified dangerous abbreviations and acronyms and symbols. Your facility may also have a list of "Do Not Use" abbreviations.

Some examples of abbreviations found to be error prone are

D/C	Discharge or discontinue
q.d. or QD	Once daily
OJ	Orange juice
TIW or tiw	3 times a week

Remember, if the person recording the information is the only one that knows what an abbreviation means, the information is useless. Others may not understand or may

---

misinterpret unapproved abbreviations. The overuse of abbreviations also can produce documentation that is not informative or useful.

E. Security of Protected Health Information

All or sections of clinical records, such as the resident assessment instrument and progress notes, may be completed by the use of computer-generated reports. Reports generated by computer software are processed and maintained in a manner to ensure the safety, integrity, and confidentiality of the clinical record.

1. Clinical Records

Protection of resident health information is a basic right for all residents. Both paper and computer information must be used in a manner that assures each resident the right to privacy. A federal law, known as the HIPAA Privacy and Security rules, governs how resident health information may be used and protected.

The clinical record is a legal document and must be stored in a manner to protect the record from loss, tampering, or unauthorized access. This means that the clinical record should not be left unattended or in areas of public access. Do not leave clinical records open when not in use.

Records that identify residents by name should be stored in locked cabinets or in a locked office when not attended. Every health care professional has a duty to protect the security of resident health information.

The original clinical record or sections of the record may not be removed from the facility. Copies of necessary information can be provided when needed by other health care providers for resident care, such as when transferring the resident to the acute hospital.

Be alert that confidential health information may appear on documents that never become part of the clinical record. Some of these documents may be schedules of appointments, flow sheets, or memoranda. All resident health information must be protected from unlawful disclosure whether part of the legal clinical record or not.

Care must be taken to dispose of resident identified papers in a manner to protect the resident's privacy. Shredders are one recommended method. Be careful when recycling papers that resident names are protected from disclosure.

2. Facsimile (FAX)

If resident health information is faxed to other caregivers, procedures need to be followed to assure privacy of information. A misdirected fax is a security breach and must be reported to administration.

- Use a fax cover sheet that identifies that the information being faxed is confidential. Provide a telephone number for the recipient to call back if the information is received in error.
- Fax machines should be located in a secure area away from public access.

- Be sure to confirm that the fax number is correct before sending the information. Use auto-dial for frequently used phone numbers to avoid misdialing errors.

3. Computers

Computers used for protected health information should be located in a secure area away from public access to protect privacy of information and prevent theft. A computer may be located at a nursing station that is off limits to residents and the public or in a private office with a locked door. Computer screens should be turned so that a passerby is unable to view the screen.

Use a personal identification code or password to access computer software. Passwords protect against unauthorized access to confidential resident health information. A password may be used only by the person to whom it is assigned. Passwords may not be shared with other personnel or consultants.

Once a user has logged on a computer program, the computer should not be left unattended. Security measures must be in place to prevent access or tampering by unauthorized users. Back up files on a regular basis to prevent loss of information.

4. E-Mail

Communicating with others about a resident's protected health information should be done with caution. HIPAA security rules require a facility to take steps to assure that e-mail is received only by the person entitled to the information. Encryption of the e-mail is not always possible, so there is risk that the information may end up in the wrong hands.

Use e-mail cautiously for communicating protected health information about a resident. At a minimum, include in the e-mail a confidentiality statement that warns a person that, if they have received this information in error, they must notify the sender.

> The following is an example of a confidentiality statement that can be included with either an e-mail or a fax of protected health information:
>
> This communication is intended solely for the addressee and is confidential. If you are not the intended recipient, any disclosure, copying, distribution, or any action taken or omitted to be taken in reliance on it, is prohibited and may be unlawful.
>
> (For Faxes) If you have received this communication in error, please notify me immediately by telephone for instructions to destroy this fax in a confidential manner.
>
> (For E-Mail) If you have received this communication in error, please notify me immediately by replying to this message and deleting it from your computer.

2. SELECTING FORMS

KEY POINTS AND SUMMARY OF CHAPTER

Activity program documentation is written on three basic kinds of forms: Assessments, Flow Sheets, and Progress Notes.

The Minimum Data Set (MDS) and a supplemental assessment form will contain the information needed to assess a resident's preferences for customary routine and activity needs.

Flow Sheet charting saves time in documenting routine activities and in finding needed information.

Follow guidelines for forms design to assure appropriate style and use.

A. Assessment Forms

Nursing facilities participating in the Medicare and Medicaid program are required to use the Resident Assessment Instrument (RAI) that includes the Minimum Data Set (MDS) and Care Area Assessments (CAAs). The MDS Section F addresses preferences for customary routine and activities. However, the MDS Section F does not contain all of the information the activity director needs to identify resident needs and strengths and develop an appropriate and individualized plan of care.

The Resident Assessment Instrument (RAI) system uses the MDS data to trigger Care Area Triggers (CATs). The activity trigger identifies residents who have or are at risk for developing adjustments to daily routines or have activity needs or problems. Residents who trigger CATs require further written assessment including decisions as to whether and how to intervene with the resident. This further information regarding the resident needs or problems is documented as a supplemental assessment in the clinical record.

Choosing and/or designing an appropriate form will make documentation easier and prevent charting errors. Well designed forms will allow efficient communication with the interdisciplinary team.

1. Types of Assessment Forms

Assessment forms used by activity professionals include:

- Minimum Data Set (MDS) Section F Preferences for Customary Routine Activities.
- Activity needs assessment form (Supplemental and/or CAA documentation)

Supplemental assessment forms are used to collect additional information about the resident's needs, strengths, preferences, and any issues that triggered the Care Area Assessment.

When selecting a supplemental assessment form, the content should include enough information to demonstrate that a CAA has been completed in the development of the activity care plan. The minimum content should include:

- Physical limitations
- Mental acuity
- Psychological well-being
- Social skills
- Spiritual needs
- Cultural values
- Accommodation of needs and special adaptations to allow participation
- Resident preferences
- Customary daily routine
- Any significant changes in activity patterns before or after admission.

2. Selecting Forms

The selection of supplemental assessment forms is based on writing style and individual preference. Paragraph style forms are suitable for narrative charting. Interventions such as activity attendance patterns are usually documented on flow sheets.

Supplemental assessments may be written:

- in a narrative format on the activity progress notes, or
- on a structured form that contains an outline of required information.

If a structured form is selected, it may simply provide an outline of topics to be assessed or it may be structured as a check off system. Some sample forms follow.

SAMPLE NURSING FACILITY
Activity Program Assessment
Page 1

Diagnosis _____ Birth Date _____

Precautions: Allergies _____ Nutrition _____

                 Mobility _____ Other _____

Customary Routines: _____

                              _____

Physical Deficits: Hearing _____

                        Vision _____

                        Dexterity _____

                        Communication _____

                        Other _____

Functional Status: Ambulatory (Self) _____

                        Assisted Ambulation _____

                        Wheelchair _____

                        Bedfast _____

                        Other _____

Mental Acuity: Alert _____

                        Oriented _____

                        Confused _____

                        Lethargic _____

                        Other _____

Social Interactions: Family _____

                        Visitors _____

                        Prefers Groups _____

                        Prefers Alone _____

                        Other _____

Psychological: Behavior _____

                        Motivation _____

                        Other _____

Religion _____ Cultural Needs _____

Language _____ Holidays_____

Resident No._____ Resident Name_____ Room No _____

Activity Program Assessment
Page 2

Recreational Preferences:

☐	Arts/Crafts	☐	Movies
☐	Bingo	☐	Music
☐	Cards	☐	Needlework
☐	Collecting	☐	Outdoors
☐	Contests	☐	Pets
☐	Cooking	☐	Sports
☐	Family	☐	Television
☐	Flower Arranging	☐	Woodworking
☐	Games	☐	Word Games
☐	Gardening	☐	Writing
☐	Group Exercises	☐	Other _____

LONG-TERM GOALS _____

_____

SHORT-TERM GOALS

☐ Increase social interaction
☐ Improve morale and sense of well-being
☐ Increase physical stamina and tolerance
☐ Increase attention span
☐ Reality orientation
☐ Stimulate imagination and decision making
☐ Develop social network and support group
☐ Sensory stimulation
☐ Other _____

PLAN:

Group Activities: _____

_____

Independent Activities: _____

_____

Family Involvement: _____

_____

DATE _____ SIGNED BY _____ A.D.

Resident No._____ Resident Name_____ Room No _____

SAMPLE NURSING FACILITY
Activity Program Assessment
Page 1

Diagnosis _____ Birth Date _____

Precautions:

Customary Routines:

Physical Deficits:

Functional Status:

Mental Acuity:

Social Interactions:

Psychological:

Religion _____ Cultural Needs _____

Language _____ Holidays_____

Resident No._____ Resident Name_____ Room No _____

Activity Program Assessment
Page 2

Recreational Preferences:

LONG-TERM GOALS

SHORT-TERM GOALS

PLAN:

Group Activities:

Independent Activities:

Family Involvement:

DATE _____ SIGNED BY _____ A.D.

Resident No._____ Resident Name_____ Room No _____

B. Flow Sheets

Flow sheet charting is a useful method of recording information about the resident in a timesaving manner. It also provides a quick method for review of information. Information is easily compared and trends spotted.

Flow sheets save time in recording and finding information. They are useful to document attendance records and one-to-one room visits.

> For example, an activity attendance record is usually a flow sheet that can be reviewed quickly to identify the resident's activity attendance pattern.
>
> Attendance information cannot be easily found if recorded in progress notes. Months of narrative progress notes would need to be read in a time consuming effort to determine if the resident had changes in activity levels.

Flow sheet charting can also be considered a type of narrative charting. If the flow sheet is designed so entries are made according to a key that is printed on the form, it is considered narrative charting. Checkmark entries are not considered narrative charting.

A combination form that includes a flow sheet and a progress note in one form can also be useful. The flow sheet can be used to document the resident's activity for a quarter. Then, at the end of the quarter, the activity director can review the resident's activity attendance and reactions. An activity progress note is written to summarize and evaluate the resident's response and participation in activity programs.

Flow sheets provide a comparative display of information for easy retrieval and evaluation. Flow sheet charting is useful for recording activity program participation simply and quickly.

C. Progress Notes

Progress notes are narrative evaluations of the resident's response to the plan of care and the progress, maintenance, or regress in respect to the goals identified in the care plan. The notes are written at the end of each quarter based on information gathered on flow sheets and from direct observation of the resident.

Usually, a plain lined form is suitable for progress notes. However, consider a form that combines a flow sheet with the progress notes. The one-to-one visit flow sheet and group activity attendance flow sheet can be combined on one side of the page. The progress note can be printed on the opposite side of the page. When the quarter has ended, the activity director simply reviews and compares the flow sheet data and writes a progress note. Once this is completed the form is placed in the clinical record.

Progress notes should to be filed in the clinical record in chronological order. This may be latest on top or in strict date order. If using the backside of a progress note for recording, strict date order works best. Keeping chart forms in the proper sequence will avoid confusion. If latest on top filing in the current record is used, three holes can be punched on both the right and left margins. When the backside of the form is used, it simply can be turned over.

SAMPLE NURSING FACILITY

Activity Attendance Record
Page 1

Month of _____ Year _____

Activity	1	2	3	4	5	6	7	8	9	10	11	12	13	14	15	16	17	18	19	20	21	22	23	24	25	26	27	28	29	30	31
Group:																															
In Room:																															
One to One:																															

Month of _____ Year _____

Activity	1	2	3	4	5	6	7	8	9	10	11	12	13	14	15	16	17	18	19	20	21	22	23	24	25	26	27	28	29	30	31
Group:																															
In Room:																															
One to One:																															

Participation Key: A: = Active   P = Passive   R = Refused

Resident No._____ Resident Name_____ Room No _____

Activity Attendance Record
Page 2

Month of _____ Year _____

Activity	1	2	3	4	5	6	7	8	9	10	11	12	13	14	15	16	17	18	19	20	21	22	23	24	25	26	27	28	29	30	31
Group:																															
In Room:																															
One to One:																															

ACTIVITY PROGRESS NOTES

Problems/Needs: _____

_____

_____

Goals/Objectives: _____

_____

_____

Response to Activity Plan: _____

_____

_____

_____

DATE _____ SIGNED BY _____ A.D.

Resident No._____ Resident Name_____ Room No _____

SAMPLE NURSING FACILITY

Activity Attendance Record
Page 1

Month of _____ Year _____

1	2	3	4	5	6	7	8	9	10	11	12	13	14	15	16	17	18	19	20	21	22	23	24	25	26	27	28	29	30	31

Month of _____ Year _____

1	2	3	4	5	6	7	8	9	10	11	12	13	14	15	16	17	18	19	20	21	22	23	24	25	26	27	28	29	30	31

Month of _____ Year _____

1	2	3	4	5	6	7	8	9	10	11	12	13	14	15	16	17	18	19	20	21	22	23	24	25	26	27	28	29	30	31

ATTENDANCE KEY

Group:		Room Visits:
A Arts / Crafts	L Movies	1 Books
B Bingo	M Music	2 Crafts
C Cards	N Needlework	3 Discussion
D Contests	O Outdoors	4 Exercises
K Cooking	P Pets	5 Games
E Exercise	S Sports	6 Music
F Flowers	T Television	7 Sensory Stimulation
G Games	U Word Games	8 Volunteer
H Gardening	W Writing	9 Family

Resident No._____   Resident Name_____ Room No _____

SAMPLE NURSING FACILITY

ACTIVITY PROGRESS NOTE

Problems/Needs: _____

_____

_____

Goals/Objectives: _____

_____

_____

Response to Activity Plan: _____

_____

_____

_____

_____

_____

_____

_____

_____

_____

_____

_____

_____

DATE _____ SIGNED BY _____ A.D.

Resident No._____ Resident Name_____ Room No _____

D. Forms Design

Whether designing a form or selecting a preprinted form, there are guidelines that will help in the selection process. Poorly designed forms can lead to charting errors. Be aware that unnecessary forms cause unnecessary paperwork.

Whenever possible, avoid duplicating any information that is already included on another form in the clinical record. Information collected in the MDS does not have to be repeated on other forms. If there is reason to make duplicate entries of information, be sure all areas agree and are not in conflict.

DESIGN GUIDELINES

- Allow ¼-inch space at top of form
- Name of facility should appear on form
- The form must have a title
- For binder systems, the left-hand margin must have ¾-inch allowance for hole punch
- Content of the forms must include a place for a date and a signature
- Space must be provided for at least the resident name, number, and room.

A pilot or testing period with a small supply of a new form is recommended. Errors and revisions are quickly spotted and can be corrected without undue expense. Corrected versions of the form are then available on a timely basis. Identify the version and revision date at the bottom of the form for control.

To avoid confusion when working with forms revision, it is helpful to include a form number and date of current revision of the form. Often multiple versions of a form circulate throughout the facility, making it difficult to determine which is the current form.

When creating a new form, it is good practice to justify the need for the form by using the following criteria:

Identify the Need:

- What purpose?
- Why the change?
- Where will it be used, filed, or stored?
- What present form does it replace?

  - Present number on hand (inventory)?

- If not replacing another form,

  - how was the information collected previously?
  - how will the new form improve the record?

Evaluate the Use:

- Who will use it?
- Procedures for completing form?

- Typed or handwritten? Computer generated?
- Estimated annual quantity?
- Compatibility and interface with other forms?

3. Resident Rights

| KEY POINTS AND SUMMARY OF CHAPTER |

The activity program is an essential part of the quality of life for residents in a nursing facility.

Activity programs are designed to promote resident dignity, enhance self-esteem and self-worth, and allow opportunities for choice, self-determination, and accommodation of the resident's special needs.

The activity professional has an obligation to maintain the confidentiality of medical or personal information about residents.

A. Resident Rights

Resident rights are the hallmark of the federal regulations governing nursing facilities. Each resident has the right to be provided care in a manner and in an environment that treats each resident as a person, recognizes each resident's individual needs, and enhances each resident's quality of life.

Quality of life depends on:

- each resident being treated with dignity and respect,
- recognition of each resident's individuality,
- allowing the resident to make choices about his or her life in the facility, and
- accommodating the resident's special needs.

B. Quality of Life

The activity program is an essential part of assuring the quality of life in the nursing facility. A well-developed activity plan with appropriate activities that are chosen based on the resident's needs, strengths, and preferences:

- maintains the resident's dignity,
- allows self-determination and accommodation of unique needs,
- enhances self-worth,
- promotes motivation and sense of well-being, and
- assists in achieving positive outcomes of care.

Quality of life is obvious through observation. Look around, see what residents are doing. Listen to the tone of conversations between staff and residents. By looking and listening it is easy to determine if staff are assuring resident rights.

Very simply, staff actions demonstrate that resident rights are respected, such as:

- Residents are well groomed and appropriately dressed.
- Staff talks and listens to residents, providing explanations to the resident when care is given.
- Residents are informed of activities that are appropriate to the resident.
- Activity programs take place according to the posted activity calendar.
- Residents are not sitting in hallways with no apparent purpose or involvement in facility daily life.
- Staff handles behavior of the residents, such as crying out, disrobing, agitation, rocking, or pacing.

Section 483.15, titled Quality of Life, contains regulations and interpretive guidelines that are instructions to surveyors on how to determine if the activity program is in compliance. The intent of these regulations is to create and sustain an environment that humanizes and individualizes the resident. The interpretive guidelines give instructions and examples for surveyors to determine if staff interactions provide residents with a sense of dignity.

CFR Section 483.15 Quality of Life

§483.15 A facility must care for its residents in a manner and in an environment that promotes maintenance or enhancement of each resident's quality of life.

(a)   Dignity.

The facility must promote care for residents in a manner and in an environment that maintains or enhances each resident's dignity, and respect in full recognition of his or her individuality.

(b)   Self-determination and participation.

The resident has the right to —

(1) Choose activities, schedules, and health care consistent with his or her interests, assessments and plans of care;
(2) Interact with members of the community both inside and outside the facility; and
(3) Make choices about aspects of his or her life in the facility that are significant to the resident.

(d)   Participation in other activities...

A resident has the right to participate in social, religious, and community

---

activities that do not interfere with the rights of other residents in the facility.

(e) **Accommodation of needs. A resident has the right to —**

(1) **Reside and receive services in the facility with reasonable accommodation of individual needs and preferences, except when the health or safety of the individual or other residents would be endangered; and**

(2) **Receive notice before the resident's room or roommate in the facility is changed.**

1. Dignity

Surveyors are instructed to observe the activity levels of residents to evaluate if residents are being treated with courtesy and respect. Dignity is observable. The manner in which staff address residents reflects dignity. Labels such as the screamer or the complainer and pet names such as Gramps, honey, sweetie are demeaning and inappropriate.

Staff should focus on the resident as an individual when talking and explain the care and/or services being provided. Staff should not have conversations in the presence of a resident that excludes his or her participation. Be careful about talking about a resident in settings within the facility where others can overhear.

Interpretive Guidelines §483.15 (a) Dignity.

"Dignity" means that in their interactions with residents, staff carries out activities that assist the resident to maintain and enhance his/her self-esteem and self-worth.

For example:

- *Grooming residents as they wish to be groomed (e.g., hair combed and styled, beards shaved/trimmed, nails clean and clipped);*

- *Encouraging and assisting residents to dress in their own clothes appropriate to the time of day and individual preferences rather than hospital-type gowns;*

- *Assisting residents to attend activities of their own choosing;*

- *Respecting resident's private space and property, e.g., not changing radio or television station without resident's permission;*

- *Knocking on doors and requesting permission to enter, closing doors as requested by the resident;*

- *Not moving or inspecting resident's personal possessions without permission;*

- *Respecting residents by speaking respectfully, addressing the resident with a name of the resident's choice, avoiding use of labels for residents such as "feeders";*

- *Not excluding residents from conversations or discussing residents in community settings in which others can overhear private information; and*

- *Focusing on residents as individuals when they talk to them and addressing residents as individuals when providing care and services.*

Procedures §483.15 (a) Dignity.

Throughout the survey, observe:

- *Do staff show respect for residents?*

- *When staff interact with a resident, do staff pay attention to the resident as an individual?*

- *Do staff respond in a timely manner to the resident's requests for assistance?*

- *In group activities, do staff focus attention on the group of residents? Or, do staff appear distracted when they interact with residents? For example, do staff continue to talk with each other while doing a task for a resident(s) as if she/he were not present?*

2. Self-determination

The activity program enhances the resident's quality of life when it includes opportunities for choice and self-determination. Whenever possible, the activity plan should allow the resident to work with the staff to set up daily schedules that consider the resident's former life style, customary routines, and personal choices. Voicing opinions, participating in resident council, making suggestions are considered empowerment activities.

Interpretive Guidelines §483.15 (b) Self-determination and Participation.

The intent of this requirement is to specify that the facility must create an environment that is respectful of the right of each resident to exercise his or her autonomy regarding what the resident considers to be important facets of his or her life. This includes actively seeking information from the resident regarding significant interests and preferences in order to provide necessary assistance to help residents fulfill their choices over aspects of their lives in the facility.

Many types of choices are mentioned in this regulatory requirement. The first of these is choice of "activities." It is an important right for a resident to have choices to participate in preferred activities, whether they are part of the formal activities program or self-directed. However, the regulation covers both formal and self-directed activities.

The second listed choice is "schedules." Resident have the right to have choice over their schedules, consistent with their interests, assessments, and plans of care. Choice over "schedules" includes (but is not limited to) choices over the schedules that are important to the resident, such as daily waking, eating, bathing, and the time for going to bed at night. Residents have the right to choose health care schedules consistent with their interests and preferences, and the facility should gather this information in order to be proactive in assisting residents to fulfill their choices. For example, if a resident mentions that her therapy is scheduled at the time of her favorite television program, the facility should accommodate the resident to the extent that it can.

Residents have the right to make choices about aspects of their lives that are significant to them. One example includes the right to choose to room with a person of the resident's choice, if both parties are residents of the facility, and both consent to the choice.

Procedures §483.15 (b) Self-determination and Participation.

- *Determine if the resident is able to exercise her/his choices regarding personal activities, including whether the facility provides assistance as needed to the resident to be able to engage in their preferred activities on a routine basis.*

- *Determine what time the resident awakens and goes to sleep, and whether this is the resident's preferred time.*

- *Determine whether the facility is honoring the resident's preferences regarding the timing (morning, afternoon, evening, and how many times a week) for bathing and also the method (shower, bath, in-bed bathing).*

- *If the resident is unaware of the right to make such choices, determine whether the facility has actively sought information from the resident and/or family (for a resident unable to express choices) regarding preferences and whether these choices have been made known to caregivers.*

The right of self-determination is intended to create a homelike environment that allows that residents to plan their daily schedules and making choices, if able. Activity staff can create and accommodate residents' special needs.

- Offer residents choices of activity programs to attend.
- If a resident refuses to attend group activities, offer one-to-one interventions and in room activities.
- If a resident has a complaint, help the resident to resolve it.
- Consider and accommodate the resident's customary routines in the resident's activity participation.
- Obtain resident and family input regarding activity choices.
- Come to know each resident and what aspects of life are important to him or her.

There is a fine line between helping a resident and taking away opportunities to make choices. Allow residents to make choices at the level of their abilities. Let the residents decide how they spend their time, both inside and outside the facility.

3. Accommodation of Needs

Many residents in nursing homes require certain accommodation to meet their unique needs. Staff may need to make adjustments to allow residents to exercise choice and self-determination. Accommodation of needs may require adaptations of environment or planned staff interventions.

> For example, accommodation of needs can be necessary for leisure activity choices, food preferences, telephone access, protection of personal property, and special accommodations for married couples.

Familiar objects and routines can provide residents with a sense of comfort and make the nursing facility feel more homelike rather than an institution. This can reduce some of the sense of loss and promote individuality. Activity staff can develop plans to accommodate a resident's needs and choices for how he/she spends time, both inside and outside the facility.

Married couples both of whom reside in the facility have the right share the same room. A spouse who resides in the community may request privacy during visits.

Interpretive Guidelines §483.15 (e) Accommodation of Needs

Reasonable accommodation of individual needs and preference is defined as the facility's efforts to individualize the resident's environment. This includes the physical environment of the resident's bedroom and bathroom, as well as individualizing as much as feasible the facility's common living areas. The facility's physical environment and staff behaviors should be directed toward assisting the resident in maintaining and/or achieving independent functioning, dignity, and well-being to the extent possible in accordance with the resident's own needs and preferences.

Procedures §483.15 (e) Accommodation of Needs

- *Observe the resident using her/his room and common areas and interview the resident if possible to determine if the environment has been adapted as necessary to accommodate the resident's needs and preferences.*

- *Observe staff/resident interactions to determine if staff members adapt their interactions so that a resident with limited sight or hearing can see and hear them. Are hearing aids and glasses in use, clean, and functional?*

- *Determine if staff use appropriate measures to facility communication with residents who have difficulty communicating. For example, do staff communicate at eye level, and do they remove a resident from noisy surroundings if that resident is having difficulty hearing what is said?*

C. Refusal

The resident's right to choice may result in resident or family refusal of activities or treatments. Offer explanations as to the rationale and importance of treatments and services but do not force residents to accept care.

Steps to take when a resident refuses care:

- treat with kindness,
- offer alternatives,
- counsel resident regarding necessity of treatment,
- report refusal to supervisor, and
- document refusal in health record.

Offer choices whenever possible:

- activities to attend,
- selection of clothing to wear,
- food preferences (likes or dislikes), or
- support comfort measures for end-of-life.

CFR Section 483.10(b)(4) Right to Refuse Treatment

§483.10(b)(4) The resident has the right to refuse treatment...

Interpretive Guidelines §483.10(b)(4) Right to Refuse Treatment

"Treatment" is defined as care provided for purposes of maintaining/restoring health, improving functional level, or relieving symptoms.

The facility should determine exactly what the resident is refusing and why. To the extent the facility is able, it should address the resident's concern... The facility is expected to assess the reasons for this resident's refusal, clarify and educate the resident as to the consequences of refusal, offer alternative treatments, and continue to provide all other services.

If a resident's refusal of treatment brings about a significant change, the facility should reassess the resident and institute care planning changes. A resident's refusal of treatment does not absolve a facility from providing a resident with care that allows him/her to maintain his/her highest practicable physical, mental, and psychosocial well-being in the context of making that refusal.

D. Privacy

The resident has the right to personal privacy and confidentiality of his or her personal and clinical records.

---

1. Personal Privacy

Resident rights provide that a resident can expect personal privacy during care and treatment. Examinations and treatments are never performed in public areas of the building. Only authorized staff directly involved in treatment should be present when treatments are given. Those not involved in the care of the individual should not be present without the resident's consent while he/she is receiving personal care or treatment.

Be aware of residents' appearance when attending activities or whenever they are in any public area of the facility. Are they dressed properly with clothing buttoned and correctly fastened? Are they sitting in a dignified manner to avoid any improper exposure? For example, use lap robes if residents are unable to sit in a modest position.

Interpretive Guidelines §483.10(e) Privacy

Right to privacy means the resident has the right to privacy with whomever the resident wishes. Privacy should include full visual, and, to the extent desired, for visits or other activities, auditory privacy. Private space may be created flexibly and need not be dedicated solely for visitation purposes.

For example, privacy for visitation or meetings might be arranged by using a dining area between meals, a vacant chapel, office, or room; or an activities area when activities are not in progress. Arrangements for private space could be accomplished through cooperation between the facility's administration and resident or family groups so that private space is provided for those requesting it without infringement on the rights of other residents.

Maintain an environment in which there are no signs posted in residents' rooms or staff work areas able to be seen by other residents and/or visitors that include confidential or personal information (such as information about incontinence, cognitive status). It is allowable to post signs with this type of information in more private locations such as the inside of a closet or in staff locations that are not viewable by the public. An exception can be made in an individual case if a resident or responsible family member insists on the posting of care information at the bedside (e.g., do not take blood pressure in right arm).

This does not prohibit the display of resident names on their doors nor does it prohibit display of resident memorabilia and/or biographical information in or outside their rooms with their consent or the consent of the responsible party if the resident is unable to give consent.

2. Confidentiality of Protected Health Information

Health care professionals are entrusted with personal health information regarding residents. This incurs an obligation and trust to maintain the confidentiality of all medical and personal information about residents. Those not involved in the care of the resident may not have access to a resident's health information unless specifically authorized by the resident or the resident's responsible person.

The Health Insurance Portability and Accountability Act (HIPAA) includes the Privacy Rule that applies to all providers of health care. These national standards protect a resident's clinical records and other personal health information.

The HIPAA Privacy Rule requires the facility to:

- Notify residents about their privacy rights and how their information can be used.
- Adopt and implement privacy procedure.
- Train employees so that they understand the privacy procedures.
- Designate a privacy officer and a security officer.
- Secure clinical records, whether in paper form or in a computer, so that they are not readily available to those who do not need them.

Do not discuss residents:

- outside of the facility (on bus going home).
- where visitors or other residents can overhear.

Resident care may be discussed:

- at interdisciplinary team conferences.
- with other health professionals.

Always be aware to whom you are speaking. Do you know that this is a person who is authorized to receive protected health information? Be aware of where you are speaking. Can those not involved in resident care overhear what you are saying?

Questions from family and friends may be answered in a general manner regarding their condition depending on their involvement with care. Questions about detailed medical treatment should be referred to the doctor or charge nurse. Such questions are answered on a need to know basis, respecting the resident's right to privacy.

Hospital elevators, hallways, and cafeterias are frequently places where staff may have conversations regarding confidential information that could be overheard. Do not discuss medical histories within earshot of strangers.

Actions that assure resident confidentiality and privacy:

- Knock on door when entering a resident's room.
- Do not leave charts open or flow sheets posted in public view.
- Do not open or read resident's mail unless requested.

Confidentiality <u>does not</u> prohibit sharing resident information among members of the health care team. To give the best possible care to the resident, all members of the health care team must be informed of the resident's condition and plan of care. Sharing information at change of shift report or at care plan conferences is not a violation of confidentiality. However, change of shift reporting and care plan conferences should be conducted in an area where other residents and visitors cannot overhear the discussion. Be aware of indiscreet conversation in public areas of the facility.

4. FEDERAL REGULATIONS

KEY POINTS AND SUMMARY OF CHAPTER

The regulations for activity programs are found in the section of the regulations titled Quality of Life.

The facility must provide an ongoing program of activities designed to accommodate the individual resident's interests and help enhance her/his physical, mental and psychosocial well-being, according to her/his comprehensive resident assessment.

Facilities are surveyed on an annual basis by state inspectors. Surveyors will observe activities, interview residents and families, and review clinical records to determine substantial compliance with regulations.

Nursing facilities participating in the Medicare and/or Medicaid programs must follow federal regulations for skilled nursing facilities. In addition, states have their own regulations. The complete text of the federal regulations developed by the Centers for Medicare and Medicaid Services (CMS) for skilled nursing facilities can be found in Section 42, Code of Federal Regulations, Part 483, et al.

CMS has converted its manuals containing regulations and guidance to surveyors from paper-based to internet-only manuals. The regulations and interpretive guidelines are found on the CMS website for their program manuals (http://www.cms.gov/Manuals). The manual that addresses skilled nursing facility regulations is the State Operations Manual (Pub 100-7). The regulations and guidelines are found in Appendix PP.

In this chapter the text of the federal regulations for the activity program is provided as well as excerpts from the CMS's instructions to surveyors on how to evaluate the facility's compliance with the regulations. The complete text of the surveyor interpretive guidelines for activities Section 483.15(f) is found in the Appendix of this book. The guidance to surveyors is not regulation but is used to assist surveyors to determine if the facility has met the regulations.

A. Activity Program

The primary goal of the activity program is to enhance the quality of the resident's life and assist the resident to achieve his or her maximum functional potential. Activity planning is a universal need for all residents.

The activity program is integrated with the comprehensive assessment and interdisciplinary care plan. The activity plan for each individual resident should complement the plans of other healthcare disciplines. Frequently activities can supplement interventions developed by other disciplines, such as exercise programs, passing nourishments, and reality orientation.

CFR Section 483.15(f)(1) Activities

§483.15(f)(1) Activities.

(1) The facility must provide for an ongoing program of activities designed to meet, in accordance with the comprehensive assessment, the interests and the physical, mental, and psychosocial well-being of each resident.

(2) The activities program must be directed by a qualified professional who

    (i) Is a qualified therapeutic recreation specialist or an activities professional who —

        (A) Is licensed or registered, if applicable, by the State in which practicing;

        (B) Is eligible for certification as a therapeutic recreation specialist or as an activities professional by a recognized accrediting body on or after October 1,1990; or

    (ii) Has 2 years of experience in a social or recreational program within the last 5 years, 1 of which was full-time in a patient activities program in a health care setting; or

    (iii) Is a qualified occupational therapist or occupational therapy assistant; or

    (iv) Has completed a training course approved by the State.

Interpretive Guidelines §483.15(f)(1) Activities

The intent of this requirement is that:

- *The facility identifies each resident's interests and needs; and*

- *The facility involves the resident in an ongoing program of activities that is designed to his or her interests and to enhance the resident's highest practicable level of physical, mental, and psychosocial well-being.*

Definitions are provided to clarify key terms used in this guidance:

- *"Activities" refer to any endeavor, other than routine ADLs, in which a resident participates that is intended to enhance her/his sense of well-being and to promote or enhance physical, cognitive, and emotional health. These include, but are not limited to, activities that promote self-esteem, pleasure, comfort, education, creativity, success, and independence.*

- *"One-to-One Programming" refers to programming provided to residents who will not or cannot effectively plan their own activity pursuits, or residents needing specialized or extended programs to enhance their overall daily routine and activity pursuit needs.*

- *"Person Appropriate" refers to the idea that each resident has a personal identity and history that involves more than just their medical illnesses or functional impairments. Activities should be relevant to the specific needs, interests, culture, background, etc. of the individual for whom they are developed.*

- *"Program of Activities" includes a combination of large and small group, one-to-one, and self-directed activities; and a system that supports the development, implementation, and evaluation of the activities provided to the residents in the facility.*

... It is important for the facility to conduct an individualized assessment of each resident to provide additional opportunities to help enhance a resident's self-esteem and dignity. Research findings and the observations of positive resident outcomes confirm that activities are an integral component of residents' lives. Residents have indicated that daily life and involvement should be meaningful. Activities are meaningful when they reflect a person's interest and lifestyle, are enjoyable to the person, help the person to feel useful, and provide a sense of belonging.

An activity plan is developed to encourage residents toward restoration of self-care and the resumption of normal activities. Activities may include hobbies or interests pursued independently by the resident, such as reading the newspaper or watching sports on television. For those who cannot realistically resume normal activities, interventions are developed to prevent further mental or physical deterioration. Activity interventions for end-of-life may include comfort measures to provide solace, spirituality, and non-drug interventions to relieve pain.

B. Activity Director Responsibilities

The activity program is directed by a qualified activity professional. Therapeutic recreation specialists, activity professionals, or occupational therapists may be certified, registered, or licensed by an organization that is a recognized accrediting body.

The activity director's responsibilities should include:

- Directing the development, implementation, supervision, and ongoing evaluation of the activity program;

- Completing the activities component of the comprehensive assessment;
- Contributing to the comprehensive care plan, goals, and approaches that are individualized to match the skills, abilities, and interest/preferences of each resident;
- Scheduling of activities, both individual and groups;
- Implementing and delegating implementation of the programs;
- Monitoring the response and reviewing/evaluating the response to the programs to determine if the activities meet the assessed needs of the resident;
- Making revisions to the activity program and to individual resident care plans as necessary.

C. Survey Process

Facilities are surveyed on an annual basis by state inspectors. The purpose of the survey is to determine if the facility is in substantial compliance with federal regulations. A review of the activity program is part of the survey process. There are two types of standard surveys depending on the state and training of the surveyors. The traditional survey is a paper-based procedure and the Quality Indicator Survey (QIS) is an electronic computer-based procedure. Both types of surveys evaluate the compliance of the nursing home.

During the standard survey process, surveyors will observe activities, interview residents and families, and review clinical records to determine:

- Compliance with residents' rights and quality of life requirements.
- The accuracy of the residents' comprehensive assessments and the adequacy of care plans based on these assessments
- The quality of services furnished, as measured by quality indicators calculated from the MDS and as self-reported by the facility.
- The effectiveness of the physical environment to empower residents, accommodate resident needs, and maintain resident safety.

The standard survey tasks are similar for both the traditional and the Quality Indicator Survey and are made up of seven tasks:

Task 1:	Off-site Survey Preparation
Task 2:	A. Entrance Conference
	B. On Site Preparatory Activities
Task 3	Initial Tour
Task 4:	Sample Selection
Task 5:	Information Gathering
	General Observations of the Facility
	Kitchen/Food Service Observation
	Resident Review

Quality of Life Assessment
Medication Pass
Quality Assessment and Assurance Review
Abuse Prohibition Review

Task 6:   Information Analysis for Deficiency Determination

Task 7:   Exit Conference

Prior to visiting a facility for survey, off-site survey preparations are completed. Surveyors review information from the State MDS database to determine the facility's unique characteristics, such as a high prevalence of young or male residents or residents with psychiatric diagnosis. From the MDS information reported, surveyors will identify concerns about the activities program meeting cultural needs, interests, and preferences.

When the surveyors arrive, an entrance conference is held with administrative staff. The survey team will request certain information they need. Also the surveyors post signs announcing that a survey is being performed and that the surveyors are available to meet in private with residents or families who have concerns. These signs are placed in areas that are easily observable by residents and visitors.

As soon as the entrance conference has been completed, surveyors will take an initial tour of the facility. During the initial tour and throughout the survey, the surveyors are instructed to observe individual, group, and bedside activities to assess the quality of the activity program. Staff may be asked to identify those residents who have no family or significant others. Based on observations during the initial tour and review of the facility characteristics reported on the MDS, the surveyors will select a sample of residents to review. Evaluation will include observation, interview, and clinical record review.

During the tour the surveyors will focus on the following:

Quality of Life:

- *Ask staff to identify those residents who have no family or significant other;*

- *Resident grooming and dress, including appropriate footwear;*

- *Staff-resident interaction related to residents' dignity; privacy and care needs, including staff availability and responsiveness to residents' requests for assistance;*

- *The way staff talk to residents, the nature and manner of interactions, and whether residents are spoken to when care is given; and*

- *Scheduled activities taking place and appropriateness to the residents.*

Emotional and behavioral conduct of the residents and the reactions and interventions by the staff:

- *Resident behaviors such as crying out, disrobing, agitation, rocking, pacing and*

- *The manner in which these behaviors are being addressed by staff, including nature and manner of staff interactions, response time, staff availability, and staff*

> *means of dealing with residents who are experiencing catastrophic reactions.*
>
> *Impact of the facility environment and safety issues:*
>
> - *Infection control practices, e.g., hand washing, glove use, and isolation procedures;*
>
> - *Functional and clean equipment, including food service equipment;*
>
> - *Presentation and maintenance of a homelike and clean environment; and*
>
> - *Availability, use, and maintenance of assistive devices.*

During information gathering, the surveyors will review clinical records, observe the activity programs, both as scheduled and those activities pursued independently by residents. Residents and families will be interviewed and asked questions regarding the care that is provided.

D. Activity Calendar

During the entrance conference the surveyors may ask to review the activity calendars for the last three months. This information must be made available within one hour of the request.

The review of the activity calendar will determine if the formal activity program:

- reflects schedules, choices, and rights of the residents,
- offers activities at hours convenient to the residents (e.g., morning, afternoon, evenings and weekends),
- reflects the cultural and religious interests of the resident population, and
- would appeal to both men and women and all age groups living in facility.

Even though surveyors may ask for the activity calendar, federal regulations do not require that an activity calendar be maintained. Local and state regulations, however, may require an activity calendar. Be sure to check local and state regulations for exact requirements. If there are no requirements and no activity calendar is maintained, inform the surveyors that a calendar is not maintained.

E. Resident Interviews

Assessment of the resident's quality of like is done by the surveyors through individual interviews, a group interview, family interviews, and observations of residents who are non-interviewable.

In a traditional survey surveyors will select or ask for assistance in selecting a sample of residents, family, and resident representatives to be interviewed. (For QIS surveys, the residents are pre-selected.) An interviewable resident is a resident who has sufficient memory and comprehension to be able to answer coherently the majority of questions contained in the Resident Interview Task. These residents should be able to make day-to-day decisions in a fairly consistent and organized manner.

The objectives of the interviews are to:

- collect information,
- verify and validate information obtained from other survey procedures, and
- provide the opportunity for all interested parties to provide what they believe is pertinent information.

Interview the resident family or resident representative, as appropriate, to determine whether:

- *The resident/representative was involved in care plan development, including defining the approaches and goals, and whether planned activities reflect preferences and choices;*

- *The resident is participating in any activities programs and, if not, the reasons for the lack of participation;*

- *The resident needs any assistance (such as setup/positioning of activity materials) or adaptation and, if so, what is needed and whether the facility is providing it to facilitate participation in activities of choice;*

- *The resident is notified of activities and offered transportation assistance as needed to the activity location within the facility or access to transportation where available and feasible to outside activities;*

- *The facility made efforts to the extent possible to accommodate the resident's choices about his/her schedule so that service provision, such as bathing and therapy services, does not routinely conflict with desired activities;*

- *The resident receives necessary equipment and supplies to complete activities;*

- *The resident receives any necessary assistance during group activities (e.g., toileting, eating assistance, ambulation assistance);*

- *Planned activity programs are occurring on a regular basis (rather than cancelled); and*

- *The resident desires activities that the facility does not provide.*

Interview activities staff as necessary to determine any of the following as pertinent to the resident:

- *What is the resident's program of activities and what are the goals;*

- *What assistance staff provide in the activities that are part of the resident's plan;*

- *How regularly the resident participates; if not participating, determine reason(s);*

- *How staff make sure the resident is informed and transported to group activities of choice;*

- *How special dietary needs and restrictions are handled during activities involving food; and*

- *How staff make sure the resident has sufficient supplies, proper lighting, and sufficient space for activities.*

F. Clinical Records

Clinical record review will assess the quality of care and quality of life that relate to the identified areas of concern for a resident. The purpose is to evaluate assessments, plans of care, and outcomes of care. The focus of the review is to determine if there has been a decline, improvement, or maintenance in resident's functional abilities.

Surveyors will review the RAI activity documentation/notes regarding the resident's activity interests, preferences, and needed adaptations. The record will be reviewed to determine whether the assessment accurately and comprehensively reflects the status of the resident. The record review of RAI information, care planning, implementation of the care plan, and evaluation of care is one element of the resident review, which determines if there has been a decline, improvement, or maintenance in identified areas.

Determine whether staff identify:

- *Longstanding interests/customary routine and how the resident's current physical, mental, and psychosocial health status affect either the resident's choice of activities or ability to participate;*

- *Specific information about how the resident prefers to participate in activities of interest (for example, if music is an interest, what kinds of music, does the resident play an instrument; if the resident listens, does the resident have the music of choice available, does the resident have the functional skills to participate independently, such as putting a CD into a player?);*

- *Any recent significant changes in activity pattern that have occurred prior to or after admission;*

- *What the resident's current need is for special adaptations in order to participate in desired activities (e.g., auditory enhancement, equipment to compensate for physical difficulties, such as use of only one hand);*

- *What needs the resident has, if any, for time limited participation (e.g., those due to short attention span, illness that permits only limited time out of bed);*

- *The resident's desired daily routine and availability of activities; and*

- *The resident's choices for group, one-to-one, and/or self-directed activities.*

- *If conditions or risks are present at the time of assessment, did the facility comprehensively assess the resident's physical, mental, and psychosocial needs to identify the risks and/or to determine underlying causes (to the extent possible) of the resident's individual activity preferences, interests, and needed adaptations, and the impact upon the resident's function, mood, and cognition?*

5. ASSESSMENT

----------- **KEY POINTS AND SUMMARY OF CHAPTER** -----------

Assessment is a coordinated process where all disciplines become involved in gathering information about the resident.

The Resident Assessment Instrument (RAI) that includes the Minimum Data Set (MDS) provides a framework for the assessment.

Section F. Preferences for Customary Routine and Activities is usually completed by the activity professional. The information is obtained directly from the resident, or through family or a significant other or staff interviews, if the resident cannot report preferences.

A. Assessment Process

The purpose of a comprehensive assessment is to identify the resident's unique strengths, needs, preferences, and potential for improvement. It allows the health professional to come to know the resident as an individual. Assessment answers the question: Who is the resident?

Comprehensive resident assessment provides the basis for development of a resident-centered care plan. Accurate and complete information sets up an environment for success. Delivery of quality health care is based on a process of gathering information about each resident in a systematic manner.

Interdisciplinary input to the assessment is gathered from various sources including the attending physician and other appropriate health professionals. Family members and the resident, if able, should be involved to identify resident preferences and family expectations.

Assessment information collected is used to develop the care plan. Once staff knows the resident, decisions are made on how best to provide care. Resident problems, preferences, special needs, and any underlying causal factors are identified. Realistic and attainable goals for each problem are developed with specific action steps to meet established goals.

Comprehensive Assessment System

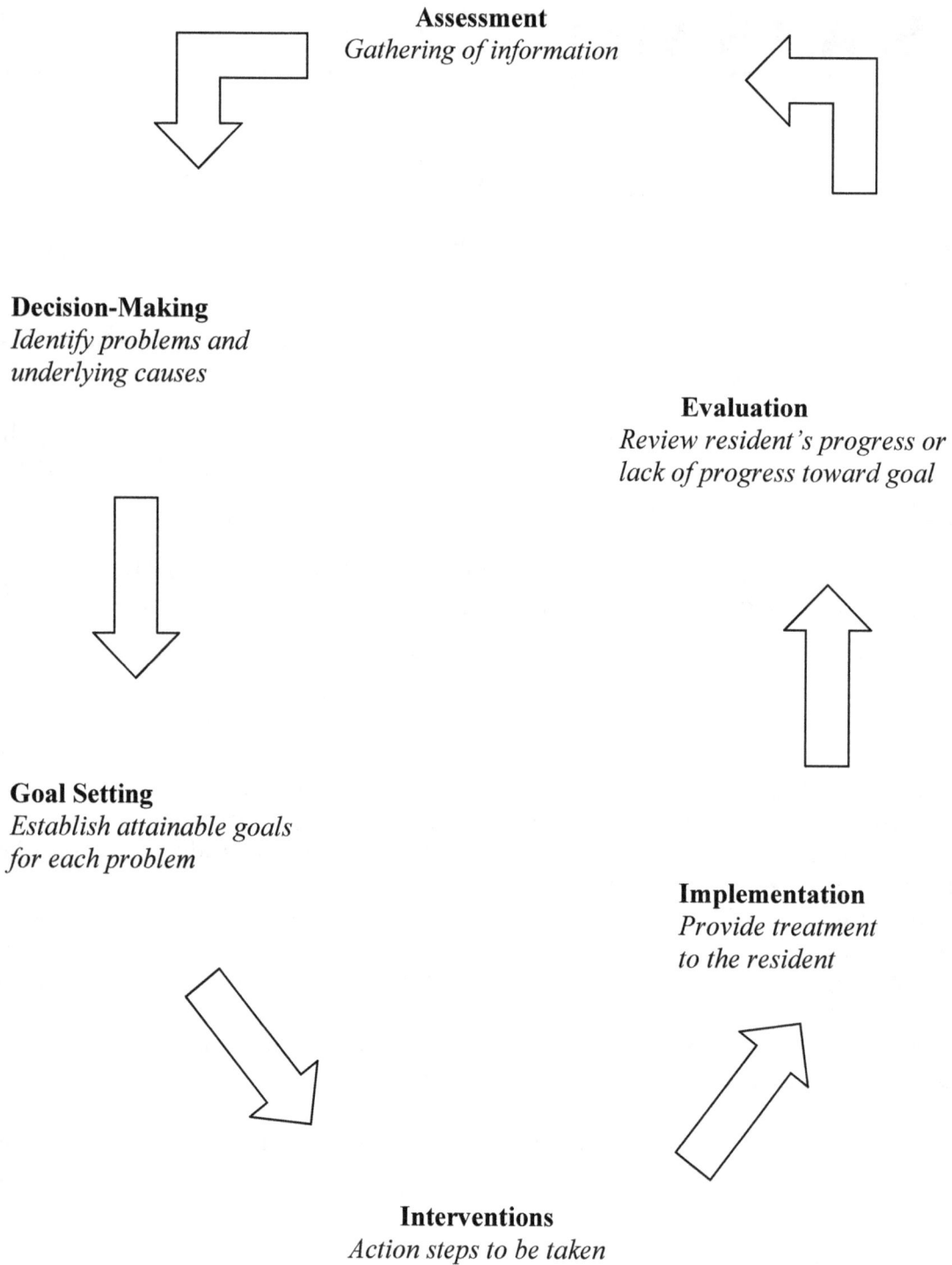

Assessment
Gathering of information

Decision-Making
*Identify problems and
underlying causes*

Evaluation
*Review resident's progress or
lack of progress toward goal*

Goal Setting
*Establish attainable goals
for each problem*

Implementation
*Provide treatment
to the resident*

Interventions
Action steps to be taken

Documentation in a SNAP

CMS Clinical Problem Solving and Decision Making Process, Steps and Objectives

Process Step / Objectives*	Key Tasks**
Recognition / Assessment *Gather essential information about the individual*	— Identify and collect information that is needed to identify an individual's conditions that enables proper definition of their conditions, strengths, needs, risks, problems, and prognosis — Obtain a personal and medical history — Perform a physical assessment
Problem definition *Define the individual's problems, risks, and issues*	— Identify any current consequences and complications of the individual's situation, underlying condition and illnesses, etc. — Clearly state the individual's issues and physical, functional, and psychosocial strengths, problems, needs, deficits, and concerns — Define significant risk factors
Diagnosis / Cause-and-effect analysis *Identify physical, functional, and psychosocial causes of risks, problems, and other issues, and how they relate to one another and to their consequences*	— Identify causes of, and factors contributing to, the individual's current dysfunctions, disabilities, impairments, and risks — Identify pertinent evaluations and diagnostic tests — Identify how existing symptoms, signs, diagnoses, test results, dysfunctions, impairments, disabilities, and other findings relate to one another — Identify how addressing those causes is likely to affect consequences
Identifying goals and objectives of care *Clarify purpose of providing care and of specific interventions, and the criteria that will be used to determine whether the objectives are being met*	— Clarify prognosis — Define overall goals for the individual — Identify criteria for meeting goals
Selecting interventions / Planning care *Identify and implement interventions and treatments to address the individual's physical, functional, and psychosocial needs, concerns, problems, and risks*	— Identify specific symptomatic and cause-specific interventions (physical, functional, and psychosocial) — Identify how current and proposed treatments and services are expected to address causes, consequences, and risk factors, and help attain overall goals for the individual — Define anticipated benefits and risks of various interventions — Clarify how specific treatments and services will be evaluated for their effectiveness and possible adverse consequences
Monitoring of progress *Review individual's progress towards goals and modify approaches as needed*	— Identify the individual's response to interventions and treatments — Identify factors that are affecting progress towards achieving goals — Define or refine the prognosis — Define or refine when to stop or modify interventions — Review effectiveness and adverse consequences related to treatments — Adjust interventions as needed — Identify when care objectives have been achieved sufficiently to allow for discharge, transfer, or change in level of care

* Refers to key steps in the care delivery process, related to clinical problem solving and decision making
** Refers to key tasks at each step in the care delivery process

Each health care discipline is responsible for implementation of the action steps in the care plan. Based on the care plan, the activity professional documents the care provided in the clinical record. Forms such as behavior monitoring records, activity attendance records, one-to-one logs, and other flow sheets contain documentation of interventions.

Periodically, a progress note is written to evaluate the care plan that describes:

- the success or lack of success in reaching the goals established in the care plan and
- resident response to the care plan.

Quarterly, each resident's care is reviewed at an interdisciplinary care conference. The resident's needs are re-evaluated. Problems, goals, and approaches are updated. If care plan goals have not been reached or the resident's condition has changed, the approaches and interventions are revised. Use resident and family input to determine realistic expected outcomes for the care plan.

B. Federal Regulations

The resident assessment instrument (RAI) developed by CMS is completed by all nursing facilities participating in Medicare and Medicaid programs. The RAI includes a Minimum Data Set (MDS) Version 3.0, the Care Area Assessment (CAA) process, and RAI utilization guidelines.

Each part of the RAI supports the comprehensive assessment process:

- The MDS is a core set of information items that have common definitions. It is a standardized data collection of assessment information for all nursing homes in the Medicare program.
- The Care Area Assessment (CAA) process identifies potential problem areas that need additional assessment to determine the need for care planning. A Care Area Trigger (CAT) identifies that the resident needs additional assessment documented in the chart. The CAA Summary form (Section V of the MDS 3.0) provides a location for documenting which CAAs have been triggered and the location in the chart where the additional assessment information can be located.
- The Utilization Guidelines provide instructions in the CMS MDS 3.0 Manual with common definitions for completion of the MDS items. These definitions must be followed when completing Section F of the MDS. In addition, clinical information is included in the federal regulations (CFR Section 483.20), known as surveyor guidance, to guide the activity professional with further assessment and development of the care plan.
- Appendix C of the MDS Users Manual provides a list of resources and tools for CAA that may be helpful, but it is not all-inclusive nor government endorsed.

Completion of the Resident Assessment Instrument (RAI) is more than a paperwork exercise. By using common, universally used definitions and coding categories, the MDS provides a systematic tool for gathering information to identify resident problems and conditions.

CFR Section 483.20 Resident Assessment

§483.20(b) Comprehensive Assessments.

(1) **Resident Assessment Instrument.** A facility must make a comprehensive assessment of a resident's needs, using the resident assessment instrument (RAI) specified by the State. The assessment must include at least the following:

    (i)   Identification and demographic information.
    (ii)   Customary routine.
    (iii)   Cognitive patterns.
    (iv)   Communication.
    (v)   Vision.
    (vi)   Mood and behavior patterns.
    (vii)   Psychological well-being.
    (viii)   Physical functioning and structural problems.
    (ix)   Continence.
    (x)   Disease diagnosis and health conditions.
    (xi)   Dental and nutritional status.
    (xii)   Skin conditions.
    (xiii)   Activity pursuit.
    (xiv)   Medications.
    (xv)   Special treatments and procedures.
    (xvi)   Discharge potential.
    (xvii)   Documentation of summary information regarding the additional assessment performed on the care areas triggered by the completion of the Minimum Data Set (MDS).
    (xviii)   Documentation of participation in assessment.

(2) When required, a facility must conduct a comprehensive assessment of a resident as follows:

    (i)   Within 14 calendar days after admission, excluding readmissions in which there is no significant change in the resident's physical or mental condition. (For purposes of this section, "readmission" means a return to the facility following a temporary absence for hospitalization or therapeutic leave.)

    (ii)   Within 14 days after the facility determines, or should have determined, that there has been a significant change in the resident's physical or mental condition. (For purpose of this section, a significant change means a major decline or improvement in the resident's status that will not normally resolve itself without further intervention by staff or by implementing standard disease-related clinical interventions, that has an impaction on more than one area of the resident's health status, and requires interdisciplinary review or revision of the care plan, or both.

(iii)   Not less than once every 12 months.

§483.20(c) Quarterly Review Assessment.

A facility must assess a resident using the quarterly review instrument specified by the State and approved by CMS not less frequently than once every 3 months.

§483.20(d) Use.

A facility must maintain all resident assessments completed within the previous 15 months in the resident's active record and use the results of the assessment to develop, review, and revise the resident's comprehensive plan of care.

§483.20(g) Accuracy of Assessment.

The assessment must accurately reflect the resident status.

§483.20(h) Coordination.

A registered nurse must conduct or coordinate each assessment with the appropriate participation of health professionals.

§483.20(i) Certification.

(1)   A registered nurse must sign and certify that the assessment is completed.

(2)   Each individual who completes a portion of the assessment must sign and certify the accuracy of that portion of the assessment.

§483.20(j) Penalty for Falsification.

(1)   Under Medicare and Medicaid, an individual who willfully and knowingly—

    (i)   Certifies a material and false statement in a resident assessment is subject to a civil money penalty of not more than $1,000 for each assessment; or

    (ii)   Causes another individual to certify a material and false statement in a resident assessment is subject to a civil money penalty of not more than $5,000 for each assessment.

Additionally, the MDS is used to determine the amount of payment for Medicare Part A Prospective Payment System and for Medicaid payment in some states. Quality monitoring by CMS uses MDS data to calculate quality indicators used in the state survey process. Using MDS data, quality measures are posted on the internet website Nursing Home Compare (http://www.medicare.gov/nhcompare/home.asp) so that consumers can access information about nursing homes. Each professional contributing must complete the MDS accurately to assure the integrity of these CMS programs.

C. Performing an Activity Needs Assessment

Activity pursuits are a need of all residents, not just those triggered by the MDS. By the very fact that the resident is in a nursing facility, their usual routines and leisure pursuits are no longer available to them. An activity needs assessment gathers information about how the resident wishes or is able to spend leisure time. The assessment should consider the residents normal everyday routines and lifetime preferences.

Promptly on admission, there must be an assessment of the resident by the activity professional to identify immediate needs. The care plan created at admission is developed to welcome the new resident, provide orientation, and ease adjustment to the facility. The assessment process starts on admission and continues throughout the resident's stay.

The purpose of assessment is to identify appropriate activity pursuits that will enhance the quality of life for each resident. The activity assessment should consider the resident's normal everyday routine and lifetime preferences. Needs and strengths are identified and incorporated into the care plan.

CFR Section 483.15(f)(1) Utilization Guidelines

The information gathered through the assessment process should be used to develop the activities component of the comprehensive care plan. The ongoing program of activities should match the skills, abilities, needs, and preferences of each resident with the demands of the activity and the characteristics of the physical, social, and cultural environments. In order to develop individualized care planning goals and approaches, the facility should obtain sufficient, detailed information (even if the Activities CAA is not triggered) to determine what activities the resident prefers and what adaptations, if any, are needed.

... The facility may use, but need not duplicate, information from other sources, such as the RAI, including the CAAs, assessments by other disciplines, observation, and resident and family interviews. Other sources of relevant information include the resident's lifelong interests, spirituality, life roles, goals, strengths, needs, and activity pursuit patterns and preferences. This assessment should be completed by or under the supervision of a qualified professional (see F249 for definition of qualified professional).

NOTE: *Some residents may be independently capable of pursuing their own activities without intervention from the facility. This information should be noted in the assessment and identified in the plan of care.*

The MDS Section F Preferences for Customary Routine and Activity is completed by a qualified activity professional. Evaluate information obtained firsthand as well as input from the interdisciplinary care team. Direct observation and interview with the resident are the first steps to gathering information. A variety of information sources may be useful and could include licensed and non-licensed staff members including nurse aides on all shifts.

Other sources of information may include, but are not limited to:

- attending physician,
- family members,
- direct care health professionals who have observed, evaluated, and/or treated the resident, and
- the clinical record, including the admission record, physician's orders, documentation of services provided to the resident, reports of any diagnostic

testing, consultation, or other services, medications administration record, copies of any transfer data provided by another health care facility, and summaries of previous discharges.

Assessment information is documented in MDS Section F and a Supplemental Activity Assessment. The MDS collects basic information, but the MDS alone does not provide a comprehensive assessment. Supplemental assessments document the decision-making process by appropriate health care professionals of the scope of the resident's problems, needs, or strengths that were triggered by the MDS. To be consistent, assessment must be made from objective and observable facts.

When assessment is performed correctly, it ensures that the plan of care is based on accurate and reliable information. A care plan based on the resident's unique needs improves the quality of life for the resident.

The activity assessment is a supplemental assessment of the resident. It includes the problems triggered by the MDS and information from the review of the Care Area Triggers (CATs) that were triggered by the MDS. This assessment utilizes information obtained not only in MDS Section F, but also from other sections of the MDS.

ELEMENTS OF A SUPPLEMENTAL ACTIVITY ASSESSMENT

1. Activity pursuit patterns, preferences, longstanding interests, and customary routines

2. How the resident's current physical, mental, and psychosocial health status affects her/his choice of activities and her/his ability to participate

3. Skills, abilities, strengths, personal goals

4. Accommodation of needs to allow participation

5. Specific information how the resident prefers to participate in activities

6. Current needs for special adaptations in order to participate in desired activities

7. Need for time-limited participation, such as short attention span or illness that permits only limited time out of bed

8. Resident's desired daily routine and availability of activities

9. Resident's choices for group, one-to-one, and self-directed activities

10. Any significant changes in activity patterns before or after admission

NOTE: Some residents may be independently capable of pursuing their own activities without intervention from the facility. This information should be noted in the assessment and identified in the care plan.

D. Resident Assessment Instrument (RAI)

By using a systematic method, the health care professional can identify problems and needs unique to each resident. The Resident Assessment Instrument (RAI), which includes the Minimum Data Set (MDS), was designed as an interdisciplinary framework to minimize duplication of effort and strengthen team communication.

1. RAI Forms

The MDS 3.0 has ten different subsets for nursing homes. Section F Preferences for Customary Routine and Activities is always contained on the comprehensive assessment form. Some states have the option to include Section F on the quarterly and PPS item sets. Check with your individual state licensing department to determine if Section F is included.

- Comprehensive (NC) Item Set. This MDS is usually called the comprehensive assessment and is done on admission, annually, for significant change in status, and for significant correction of prior comprehensive assessments.
- Quarterly (NQ) Item Set. This MDS is usually called the quarterly assessment. It is done at ninety-day intervals between annual comprehensive assessments. The quarterly MDS may be a stand-alone assessment or may be combined with another scheduled assessment such as a scheduled PPS assessment, OMRA assessment, or a discharge assessment.
- PPS (NP) Item Set. This MDS is usually called a Medicare Assessment (Prospective Payment System, PPS). Medicare Part A assessments are done during the resident Medicare covered stay at 5-day, 14-day, 30-day, 60-day, or 90-day.

2. Assessment Reference Date

Item A2300 Assessment Reference Date (ARD) of the MDS is used to establish a common reference point for all data reported in the MDS. The assessment reference date (ARD) it is the last day of the period of time that the MDS assessment covers for that particular assessment for that particular resident. Since a day begins at 12:00 AM and ends at 11:59 PM, that ARD must also cover this time period.

The ARD is scheduled by the RN Coordinator to assure that all items on the MDS reflect information from same period of time. The ARD also "drives" the due date of the next assessment. For example, the next comprehensive assessment is due within 366 days after the ARD of the most recent comprehensive assessment.

3. Time Frames

MDS scheduling will be done by the RN Coordinator. Activity professionals need to make sure they receive communication of the MDS schedule to assure timely input.

At least annually or if the resident experiences significant change, a comprehensive assessment instrument must be redone. This includes MDS, Care Area Triggers, and Care Area Assessment. Each resident must have a comprehensive resident assessment no later than 366 days following the last comprehensive assessment. Some states may have additional requirements for the MDS completion.

Should a resident be transferred to an acute hospital and then return to the facility, the RN Coordinator will determine if the resident has had a significant change in condition.

MDS SCHEDULE	
Type of Assessment	**Timing of Assessment**
Admission Assessment (Initial)	Must be completed by the 14th day of the resident's stay. The day of admission is counted as Day 1.
Annual Reassessment	Must be completed within 366 days of the most recent comprehensive assessment and within 92 days of the last quarterly assessment.
Significant Change in Status Reassessment	Must be completed by the end of the 14th calendar day following determination that a significant change has occurred

A new comprehensive assessment is completed if the resident has experienced a significant change in status.

Do not conduct another assessment if the resident is readmitted and there has not been a significant change. However, for all readmissions, the immediate long-term or short-term activity needs must be re-evaluated even though there is no significant change.

4. Quarterly Review Assessment

Each resident's activity status is reviewed quarterly. Even though MDS Section F is not part of every quarterly MDS form (depending on the state), the activity professional is part of the interdisciplinary team and must actively participate in the quarterly review. Many data items usually addressed in MDS Section F affect the resident's activity pursuits and need to be reviewed.

Interpretive Guidelines Section 483.20(c) Quarterly Review Assessment

Intent: To assure that the resident's assessment is updated on at least a quarterly basis.

At least each quarter, the facility shall review each resident with respect to those MDS items specified under the States' quarterly review requirement. At a minimum, this would include all items contained in CMS' standard quarterly review form. A Quarterly review assessment must be completed within 92 days of the ARD of the most recent clinical assessment. If the resident has experienced a significant change in status, the next quarterly review is due no later than 3 months after the ARD of the significant change reassessment.

- *Is the facility assessing and acting, no less than once every 3 months, on the results of resident's functional and cognitive status examinations?*

- *Is the quarterly review of the resident's condition consistent with information in the progress notes, the plan of care, and your (surveyor) resident observations and reviews?*

Comparison of quarterly assessment areas will assist with identifying any decline or improvement in a resident's functioning. If changes within the data elements indicate significant change, a comprehensive RAI must be completed for the resident within fourteen (14) days.

If there have been changes in the resident's status that are not considered significant change, the appropriateness of the care plan is assessed. Goals are reviewed to determine if they are still realistic for the resident. If appropriate, changes in approaches and interventions are made to assist the resident to achieve the care plan goals.

5. Significant Change of Condition MDS

Each resident is examined and reassessed with the quarterly MDS. A comparison is made at this time to determine if there has been a significant change in condition of the resident that would require a new comprehensive MDS assessment under the regulations for significant change. As part of the interdisciplinary team, activity professionals must be alert to indicators of significant change.

> *CMS's RAI Version 3.0 Manual states that a "significant change" is a decline or improvement in a resident's status that:*
>
> - *Will not normally resolve itself without intervention by staff or by implementing standard disease-related clinical interventions, is not "self-limiting" (for declines only).*
>
> - *Impacts more than one area of the resident's health status; and*
>
> - *Requires interdisciplinary review and/or revision of the care plan.*

Some indicators of significant change may include, but are not limited to, any of the following, or may be determined by a physician's decision, if uncertainty exists:

- Resident's decision making changes. (Consider whether activity programs are suitable for resident's cognitive level.)
- Emergence of a mood pattern not previously reported by the resident or staff. (Perhaps resulting in refusal to attend activity programs).
- Increase in the frequency of behavioral symptoms. (i.e., an increase in disruptive behavior).
- Begin to use trunk restraint or a chair that prevents rising for a resident when it was not used before.
- Emergence of a condition/disease in which a resident is judged to be unstable.
- Overall deterioration or improvement of resident condition.
- When a terminally ill resident enrolls in a hospice program and remains a resident at the nursing home. This is to ensure that a coordinated plan of care between the hospice and the nursing home is in place.

For example, Mr. T no longer responds to verbal requests to alter his screaming behavior. It now occurs daily and has neither lessened on its own nor responded to treatment. He is also starting to resist his daily care, pushing staff away from him as they attempt to assist with his ADLs. The resident also has started to become disruptive in group activity programs.

This is a significant change and reassessment is required since there has been deterioration in the behavioral symptoms to the point where it is occurring daily and new approaches are needed to alter the behavior. Mr. T's behavioral symptoms could have many causes, and reassessment will provide an opportunity for staff to consider illness, medication reactions, environmental stress, and other possible sources of Mr. T's disruptive behavior.

The following are not considered significant changes:

- Discrete and easily reversible causes for which the facility staff can initiate corrective action.
- Short-term illness from which staff expects a full recovery.
- Well established, predictive cyclical patterns of clinical signs and symptoms with previously diagnosed conditions.
- If the resident continues to make steady progress under the current course of care, reassessment is required only when the condition has stabilized. However, if the facility is engaged in discharge planning, a reassessment is not required.
- In an end-stage disease status (except for hospice enrollment MDS), a full reassessment would depend on a clinical determination of whether the symptoms or condition are an expected course of deterioration or not.

E. Interviewing in MDS Assessments

Information for Section F Preferences for Customary Routine and Activities is collected by interview with the resident, if able to communicate, or with a family member or significant other. If the resident is rarely/never understood and family/significant other is not available, the activity professional will make the assessment based on observations and input from the interdisciplinary team.

All residents capable of any communication should be asked to provide information regarding what they consider to be the most important facets of their lives. Self-report is the single most reliable indicator of these topics. Appendix D of the CMS's RAI Version 3.0 Manual contains a resource for interviewing to increase a resident's voice in MDS assessment.

There are some basic approaches that can make interviews simpler and more effective:

- Introduce yourself to the resident.
- Be sure the resident can hear what you are saying.
- Ask whether the resident would like an interpreter (language or signing).
- Find a quiet, private area where you are not likely to be interrupted or overheard.
- Sit where the resident can see you clearly and you can see his or her expressions.
- Establish rapport and respect.
- Explain the purpose of the question to the resident.
- Say and show the item responses.

- Ask the questions as they appear in the questionnaire.
- Break the question apart if necessary.
- Clarify by echoing what they told you.
- Repeat the response options as needed.
- Move on to another question if the resident is unable to answer.
- Break up the interview if the resident becomes tired or needs to leave for rehabilitation, etc.
- Do not try to talk a resident out of an answer.
- Record the resident's response, not what you believe they should have said.
- If the resident becomes deeply sorrowful or agitated, sympathetically respond to his or her feelings.
- Resident preferences may be influenced by many factors in a resident's physical, psychological, and environment state, and can be challenging to truly discern.

Section F of the MDS is shown on the next two pages.

Section F	Preferences for Customary Routine and Activities

F0300. Should Interview for Daily and Activity Preferences be Conducted? - Attempt to interview all residents able to communicate. If resident is unable to complete, attempt to complete interview with family member or significant other

Enter Code
☐
   0. **No** (resident is rarely/never understood <u>and</u> family/significant other not available) → Skip to and complete F0800, Staff Assessment of Daily and Activity Preferences
   1. **Yes** → Continue to F0400, Interview for Daily Preferences

---

F0400. Interview for Daily Preferences

Show resident the response options and say: **"While you are in this facility..."**

Coding:
1. **Very important**
2. **Somewhat important**
3. **Not very important**
4. **Not important at all**
5. **Important, but can't do or no choice**
9. **No response or non-responsive**

↓ Enter Codes in Boxes

☐ A. how important is it to you to **choose what clothes to wear?**

☐ B. how important is it to you to **take care of your personal belongings or things?**

☐ C. how important is it to you to **choose between a tub bath, shower, bed bath, or sponge bath?**

☐ D. how important is it to you to **have snacks available between meals?**

☐ E. how important is it to you to **choose your own bedtime?**

☐ F. how important is it to you to **have your family or a close friend involved in discussions about your care?**

☐ G. how important is it to you to **be able to use the phone in private?**

☐ H. how important is it to you to **have a place to lock your things to keep them safe?**

F0500. Interview for Activity Preferences

Show resident the response options and say: **"While you are in this facility..."**

Coding:
1. **Very important**
2. **Somewhat important**
3. **Not very important**
4. **Not important at all**
5. **Important, but can't do or no choice**
9. **No response or non-responsive**

↓ Enter Codes in Boxes

☐ A. how important is it to you to **have books, newspapers, and magazines to read?**

☐ B. how important is it to you to **listen to music you like?**

☐ C. how important is it to you to **be around animals such as pets?**

☐ D. how important is it to you to **keep up with the news?**

☐ E. how important is it to you to **do things with groups of people?**

☐ F. how important is it to you to **do your favorite activities?**

☐ G. how important is it to you to **go outside to get fresh air when the weather is good?**

☐ H. how important is it to you to **participate in religious services or practices?**

F0600. Daily and Activity Preferences Primary Respondent

Enter Code
☐
Indicate primary respondent for Daily and Activity Preferences (F0400 and F0500)
   1. **Resident**
   2. **Family or significant other** (close friend or other representative)
   9. **Interview could not be completed** by resident or family/significant other ("No response" to 3 or more items)

MDS 3.0 Nursing Home Comprehensive (NC) Version 1.10.3 Effective 04/01/2012

Section F	Preferences for Customary Routine and Activities

F0700. Should the Staff Assessment of Daily and Activity Preferences be Conducted?

<table>
<tr>
<td>Enter Code
☐</td>
<td>0. No (because Interview for Daily and Activity Preferences (F0400 and F0500) was completed by resident or family/significant other) → Skip to and complete G0110, Activities of Daily Living (ADL) Assistance
1. Yes (because 3 or more items in Interview for Daily and Activity Preferences (F0400 and F0500) were not completed by resident or family/significant other) → Continue to F0800, Staff Assessment of Daily and Activity Preferences</td>
</tr>
</table>

F0800. Staff Assessment of Daily and Activity Preferences

Do not conduct if Interview for Daily and Activity Preferences (F0400-F0500) was completed

Resident Prefers:

↓ Check all that apply

- ☐ A. Choosing clothes to wear
- ☐ B. Caring for personal belongings
- ☐ C. Receiving tub bath
- ☐ D. Receiving shower
- ☐ E. Receiving bed bath
- ☐ F. Receiving sponge bath
- ☐ G. Snacks between meals
- ☐ H. Staying up past 8:00 p.m.
- ☐ I. Family or significant other involvement in care discussions
- ☐ J. Use of phone in private
- ☐ K. Place to lock personal belongings
- ☐ L. Reading books, newspapers, or magazines
- ☐ M. Listening to music
- ☐ N. Being around animals such as pets
- ☐ O. Keeping up with the news
- ☐ P. Doing things with groups of people
- ☐ Q. Participating in favorite activities
- ☐ R. Spending time away from the nursing home
- ☐ S. Spending time outdoors
- ☐ T. Participating in religious activities or practices
- ☐ Z. None of the above

Uniform guidelines have been developed by CMS for completing the MDS. Because this system is used nationwide, it is important that health professionals use the same definitions and methods to collect data.

In most facilities, an activity professional will be responsible for completing Section F. Follow the MDS definitions carefully. Do not make up or change definitions.

SECTION F: PREFERENCES FOR CUSTOMARY ROUTINE AND ACTIVITIES

Intent

The intent of items in this section is to obtain information regarding the resident's preferences for his or her daily routine and activities. This is best accomplished when the information is obtained directly from the resident or through family or significant other, or staff interviews if the resident cannot report preferences. The information obtained during this interview is just a portion of the assessment. Nursing homes should use this as a guide to create an individualized plan based on the resident's preferences, and is not meant to be all-inclusive.

F0300: Should Interview for Daily and Activity Preferences Be Conducted?

Item Rationale

Health-related Quality of Life

- Most residents capable of communicating can answer questions about what they like.
- Obtaining information about preferences directly from the resident, sometimes called "hearing the resident's voice," is the most reliable and accurate way of identifying preferences.
- If a resident cannot communicate, then family or significant other who knows the resident well may be able to provide useful information about preferences.

Planning for Care

- Quality of life can be greatly enhanced when care respects the resident's choice regarding anything that is important to the resident.
- Interviews allow the resident's voice to be reflected in the care plan.
- Information about preferences that comes directly from the resident provides specific information for individualized daily care and activity planning.

Steps for Assessment

1. Determine whether or not resident is rarely/never understood and if family/significant other is available. If resident is rarely/never understood and family is not available, skip to item F0800, Staff Assessment of Daily and Activity Preferences.
2. Review Language item (A1100) to determine whether or not the resident needs or wants an interpreter.

- If the resident needs or wants an interpreter, complete the interview with an interpreter.

3. The resident interview should be conducted if the resident can respond:
   - verbally,
   - by pointing to their answers on the cue card, OR
   - by writing out their answers.

Coding Instructions

Record whether the resident preference interview should be attempted.

- **Code 0, no:** if the interview should not be attempted with the resident. This option should be selected for residents who are rarely/never understood, who need an interpreter but one was not available, and who do not have a family member or significant other available for interview. Skip to F0800, (Staff Assessment of Daily and Activity Preferences).
- **Code 1, yes:** if the resident interview should be attempted. This option should be selected for residents who are able to be understood, for whom an interpreter is not needed or is present, or who have a family member or significant other available for interview. Continue to F0400 (Interview for Daily Preferences) and F0500 (Interview for Activity Preferences).

Coding Tips and Special Populations

- If the resident needs an interpreter, every effort should be made to have an interpreter present for the MDS clinical interview. If it is not possible for a needed interpreter to be present on the day of the interview, and a family member or significant other is not available for interview, code F0300 = 0 to indicate interview not attempted, and complete the Staff Assessment of Daily and Activity Preferences (F0800) instead of the interview with the resident (F0400 and F0500).

F0400: Interview for Daily Preferences

Item Rationale

Health-related Quality of Life

- Individuals who live in nursing homes continue to have distinct lifestyle preferences.
- A lack of attention to lifestyle preferences can contribute to depressed mood and increased behavior symptoms.
- Resident responses that something is important but that they can't do it or have no choice can provide clues for understanding pain, perceived functional limitations, and perceived environmental barriers.

Planning for Care

- Care planning should be individualized and based on the resident's preferences.
- Care planning and care practices that are based on resident preferences can lead to
  — improved mood,
  — enhanced dignity, and

— increased involvement in daily routines and activities.

- Incorporating resident preferences into care planning is a dynamic, collaborative process. Because residents may adjust their preferences in response to events and changes in status, the preference assessment tool is intended as a first step in an ongoing dialogue between care providers and the residents. Care plans should be updated as residents' preferences change, paying special attention to preferences that residents state are important.

Steps for Assessment: Interview Instructions

1. Interview any resident not screened out by the "Should Interview for Daily and Activity Preferences Be Conducted?" item (F0300).
2. Conduct the interview in a private setting.
3. Sit so that the resident can see your face. Minimize glare by directing light sources away from the resident's face.
4. Be sure the resident can hear you.

- Residents with hearing impairment should be interviewed using their usual communication devices/techniques, as applicable.
- Try an external assistive device (headphones or hearing amplifier) if you have any doubt about hearing ability.
- Minimize background noise.

5. Explain the reason for the interview before beginning.

Suggested language: "I'd like to ask you a few questions about your daily routines. The reason I'm asking you these questions is that the staff here would like to know what's important to you. This helps us plan your care around your preferences so that you can have a comfortable stay with us. Even if you're only going to be here for a few days, we want to make your stay as personal as possible."

6. Explain the interview response choices. While explaining, also show the resident a clearly written list of the response options, for example a cue card.

Suggested language: "I am going to ask you how important various activities and routines are to you while you are in this home. I will ask you to answer using the choices you see on this card [read the answers while pointing to cue card]: 'Very Important,' 'Somewhat important,' 'Not very important,' 'Not important at all,' or 'Important, but can't do or no choice.'"

Explain the "Important, but can't do or no choice" response option.

Suggested language: "Let me explain the 'Important, but can't do or no choice' answer. You can select this answer if something would be important to you, but because of your health or because of what's available in this nursing home, you might not be able to do it. So, if I ask you about something that is important to you, but you don't think you're able to do it now, answer 'Important, but can't do or no choice.' If you choose this option, it will help us to think about ways we might be able to help you do those things."

7. Residents may respond to questions

- verbally,

- by pointing to their answers on the cue card, OR
- by writing out their answers.

8. If resident cannot report preferences, then interview family or significant others.

Coding Instructions

- **Code 1, very important:** if resident, family, or significant other indicates that the topic is "very important."
- **Code 2, somewhat important:** if resident, family, or significant other indicates that the topic is "somewhat important."
- **Code 3, not very important:** if resident, family, or significant other indicates that the topic is "not very important."

> **DEFINITIONS**
>
> **NONSENSICAL RESPONSE**
> Any unrelated, incomprehensible, or incoherent response that is not informative with respect to the item being rated.

- **Code 4, not important at all:** if resident, family, or significant other indicates that the topic is "not important at all."
- **Code 5, important, but can't do or no choice:** if resident, family, or significant other indicates that the topic is "important," but that he or she is physically unable to participate, or has no choice about participating while staying in nursing home because of nursing home resources or scheduling.
- **Code 9, no response or non-responsive:**

  — If resident, family, or significant other refuses to answer or says he or she does not know.
  — If resident does not give an answer to the question for several seconds and does not appear to be formulating an answer.
  — If resident provides an incoherent or nonsensical answer that does not correspond to the question.

Coding Tips and Special Populations

- The interview is considered incomplete if the resident gives nonsensical responses or fails to respond to 3 or more of the 16 items in F0400 and F0500. If the interview is stopped because it is considered incomplete, fill the remaining F0400 and F0500 items with a 9 and proceed to F0600, Daily Activity Preferences Primary Respondent.
- No look-back is provided for resident. He or she is being asked about current preferences while in the nursing home but is not limited to a 7-day look-back period to convey what their preferences are.
- The facility is still obligated to complete the assessment within the 7-day look-back period.

Interviewing Tips and Techniques

- Sometimes respondents give long or indirect answers to interview items. To narrow the answer to the response choices available, it can be useful to summarize their longer answer and then ask them which response option best applies. This is known as echoing.

- For these questions, it is appropriate to explore residents' answers and try to understand the reason.

Examples for F0400A, How Important Is It to You to Choose What Clothes to Wear (including hospital gowns or other garments provided by the facility)?

1. Resident answers, "It's very important. I've always paid attention to my appearance."

   Coding: F0400A would be **coded 1, very important**.

2. Resident replies, "I leave that up to the nurse. You have to wear what you can handle if you have a stiff leg."

   Interviewer echoes, "You leave it up to the nurses. Would you say that, while you are here, choosing what clothes to wear is [pointing to cue card] very important, somewhat important, not very important, not important at all, or that it's important, but you can't do it because of your leg?"

   Resident responds, "Well, it would be important to me, but I just can't do it."

   Coding: F0400A would be **coded 5, important, but can't do or no choice**.

Examples for F0400B, How Important Is It to You to Take Care of Your Personal Belongings or Things?

1. Resident answers, "It's somewhat important. I'm not a perfectionist, but I don't want to have to look for things."

   Coding: F0400B would be **coded 2, somewhat important**.

2. Resident answers, "All my important things are at home."

> DEFINITIONS:
>
> **PERSONAL BELONGINGS OR THINGS**
> Possessions such as eyeglasses, hearing aids, clothing, jewelry, books, toiletries, knickknacks, pictures.

   Interviewer clarifies, "Your most important things are at home. Do you have any other things while you're here that you think are important to take care of yourself?"

   Resident responds, "Well, my son brought me this CD player so that I can listen to music. It is very important to me to take care of that."

   Coding: F0400B would be **coded 1, very important**.

Examples for F0400C, How Important Is It to You to Choose between a Tub Bath, Shower, Bed Bath, or Sponge Bath?

1. Resident answers, "I like showers."

   Interviewer clarifies, "You like showers. Would you say that choosing a shower instead of other types of bathing is very important, somewhat important, not very important, not important at all, or that it's important, but you can't do it or have no choice?"

   The resident responds, "It's very important."

   Coding: F0400C would be **coded 1, very important**.

2. Resident answers, "I don't have a choice. I like only sponge baths, but I have to take shower two times a week."

   The interviewer says, "So how important is it to you to be able to choose to have a sponge bath while you're here?"

   The resident responds, "Well, it is very important, but I don't always have a choice because that's the rule."

   Coding: F0400C would be **coded 5, important, but can't do or no choice**.

> DEFINITIONS:
>
> **BED BATH**
> Bath taken in bed using washcloths and water basin or other method in bed.
>
> **SHOWER**
> Bath taken standing or using gurney or shower chair in a shower room or stall.
>
> **SPONGE BATH**
> Bath taken sitting or standing at sink.
>
> **TUB BATH**
> Bath taken in bathtub.

Example for F0400D, How Important Is It to You to Have Snacks Available between Meals?

1. Resident answers, "I'm a diabetic, so it's very important that I get snacks."

   Coding: F0400D would be **coded 1, very important**.

> DEFINITIONS:
>
> **SNACK**
> Food available between meals, including between dinner and breakfast.

Example for F0400E, How Important Is It to You to Choose Your Own Bedtime?

1. Resident answers, "At home I used to stay up and watch TV. But here I'm usually in bed by 8. That's because they get me up so early."

Interviewer echoes and clarifies, "You used to stay up later, but now you go to bed before 8 because you get up so early. Would you say it's [pointing to cue card] very important, somewhat important, not very important, not important at all, or that it's important, but you don't have a choice about your bedtime?"

Resident responds, "I guess it would be important, but I can't do it because they wake me up so early in the morning for therapy and by 8 o'clock at night, I'm tired."

Coding: F0400E would be **coded 5, important, but can't do or no choice**.

Example for F0400F, How Important Is It to You to Have Your Family or a Close Friend Involved in Discussions about Your Care?

1. Resident responds, "They're not involved. They live in the city. They've got to take care of their own families."

    Interviewer replies, "You said that your family and close friends aren't involved right now. When you think about what you would prefer, would you say that it's very important, somewhat important, not very important, not important at all, or that it is important but you have no choice or can't have them involved in decisions about your care?"

    Resident responds, "It's somewhat important."

    Coding: F0400F would be **coded 2, somewhat important**.

Example for F0400G, How Important Is It to You to Be Able to Use the Phone in Private?

1. Resident answers, "That's not a problem for me, because I have my own room. If I want to make a phone call, I just shut the door."

DEFINITIONS:
PRIVATE TELEPHONE CONVERSATION A telephone conversation on which no one can listen in, other than the resident.

    Interviewer echoes and clarifies, "So, you can shut your door to make a phone call. If you had to rate how important it is to be able to use the phone in private, would you say it's very important, somewhat important, not very important, or not important at all?"

    Resident responds, "Oh, it's very important."

    Coding: F0400G would be **coded 1, very important**.

Example for F0400H, How Important Is It to You to Have a Place to Lock Your Things to Keep Them Safe?

1. Resident answers, "I have a safe deposit box at my bank, and that's where I keep family heirlooms and personal documents."

   Interviewer says, "That sounds like a good service. While you are staying here, how important is it to you to have a drawer or locker here?"

   Resident responds, "It's not very important. I'm fine with keeping all my valuables at the bank."

   Coding: F0400H would be **coded 3, not very important**.

F0500: Interview for Activity Preferences

Item Rationale

Health-related Quality of Life

- Activities are a way for individuals to establish meaning in their lives, and the need for enjoyable activities and pastimes does not change on admission to a nursing home.
- A lack of opportunity to engage in meaningful and enjoyable activities can result in boredom, depression, and behavior disturbances.
- Individuals vary in the activities they prefer, reflecting unique personalities, past interests, perceived environmental constraints, religious and cultural background, and changing physical and mental abilities.

Planning for Care

- These questions will be useful for designing individualized care plans that facilitate residents' participation in activities they find meaningful.
- Preferences may change over time and extend beyond those included here. Therefore, the assessment of activity preferences is intended as a first step in an ongoing informal dialogue between the care provider and resident.
- As with daily routines, responses may provide insights into perceived functional, emotional, and sensory support needs.

Coding Instructions

- See Coding Instructions for daily preferences. Coding approach is identical to that for daily preferences.

Coding Tips and Special Populations

- See Coding Tips for daily preferences Coding tips include those for daily preferences.
- Include Braille and or audio-recorded material when coding items in F0500A.

<u>Interviewing Tips and Techniques</u>

- See Interview Tips and Techniques for daily preferences
- Coding tips and techniques are identical to those for daily preferences.

<u>Examples for F0500A, How Important Is It to You to Have Books (Including Braille and Audio-recorded Format), Newspapers, and Magazines to Read?</u>

1. Resident answers, "Reading is very important to me."

   Coding: F0500A would be **coded 1, very important**.

2. Resident answers, "They make the print so small these days. I guess they are just trying to save money."

   Interviewer replies, "The print is small. Would you say that having books, newspapers, and magazines to read is very important, somewhat important, not very important, not important at all, or that it is important but you can't do it because the print is so small?"

   Resident answers: "It would be important, but I can't do it because of the print."

   Coding: F0500A would be **coded 5, important, but can't do or no choice**.

DEFINITIONS
READ Script, Braille, or audio-recorded written material.
NEWS News about local, state, national, or international current events.
KEEP UP WITH THE NEWS Stay informed by reading, watching, or listening.
NEWSPAPERS AND MAGAZINE Any type, such as journalistic, professional, and trade publications in script, Braille, or audio-recorded format.

<u>Example for F0500B, How Important Is It to You to Listen to Music You Like?</u>

1. Resident answers, "It's not important, because all we have in here is TV. They keep it blaring all day long."

   Interviewer echoes, "You've told me it's not important because all you have is a TV. Would you say it's not very important or not important at all to you to listen to music you like while you are here? Or are you saying that it's important, but you can't do it because you don't have a radio or CD player?"

   Resident responds, "Yeah. I'd enjoy listening to some jazz if I could get a radio."

Coding: F0500B would be **coded 5, important, but can't do or no choice**.

Examples for F0500C, How Important Is It to You to Be Around Animals Such as Pets?

1. Resident answers, "It's very important for me NOT to be around animals. You get hair all around and I might inhale it."

   Coding: F0500C would be **coded 4, not important at all**.

2. Resident answers, "I'd love to go home and be around my own animals. I've taken care of them for years and they really need me."

   Interviewer probes, "You said you'd love to be at home with your own animals. How important is it to you to be around pets while you're staying here? Would you say it is [points to card] very important, somewhat important, not very important, not important at all, or is it important, but you can't do it or don't have a choice about it."

   Resident responds, "Well, it's important to me to be around my own dogs, but I can't be around them. I'd say important but can't do."

   Coding: F0500C would be **coded 5, Important, but can't do or no choice**.

   Rationale: Although the resident has access to therapeutic dogs brought to the nursing home, he does not have access to the type of pet that is important to him.

Example for F0500D, How Important Is It to You to Keep Up with the News?

1. Resident answers, "Well, they are all so liberal these days, but it's important to hear what they are up to."

   Interviewer clarifies, "You think it is important to hear the news. Would you say it is [points to card] very important, somewhat important, or it's important but you can't do it or have no choice?"

   Resident responds, "I guess you can mark me somewhat important on that one."

   Coding: F0500D would be **coded 2, somewhat important**.

Example for F0500E, How Important Is It to You to Do Things with Groups of People?

1. Resident answers, "I've never really liked groups of people. They make me nervous."

    Interviewer echoes and clarifies, "You've never liked groups. To help us plan your activities, would you say that while you're here, doing things with groups of people is very important, somewhat important, not very important, not important at all, or would it be important to you but you can't do it because you feel nervous about it?"

    Resident responds, "At this point I'd say it's not very important."

    Coding: F0500E would be **coded 3, not very important**.

Examples for F0500F, How Important Is It to You to Do Your Favorite Activities?

1. Resident answers, "Well, it's very important, but I can't really do my favorite activities while I'm here. At home, I used to like to play board games, but you need people to play and make it interesting. I also like to sketch, but I don't have the supplies I need to do that here. I'd say important but no choice."

    Coding: F0500F would be **coded 5, important, but can't do or no choice**.

2. Resident answers, "I like to play bridge with my bridge club."

    Interviewer probes, "Oh, you like to play bridge with your bridge club. How important is it to you to play bridge while you are here in the nursing home?"

    Resident responds, "Well, I'm just here for a few weeks to finish my rehabilitation. It's not very important."

    Coding: F0500F would be **coded 3, not very important**.

Example for F0500G, How Important Is It to You to Go Outside to Get Fresh Air When the Weather Is Good (Includes Less Temperate Weather if Resident Has Appropriate Clothing)?

1. Resident answers, "They have such a nice garden here. It's very important to me to go out there."

    Coding: F0500G would be **coded 1, very important**.

DEFINITIONS:

OUTSIDE
Any outdoor area in the proximity of the facility, including patio, porch, balcony, sidewalk, courtyard, or garden

Examples for F0500H, How Important Is It to You to Participate in Religious Services or Practices?

1. Resident answers, "I'm Jewish. I'm Orthodox, but they have Reform services here. So I guess it's not important."

    Interviewer clarifies, "You're Orthodox, but the services offered here are Reform. While you are here, how important would it be to you to be able to participate in religious services? Would you say it is very important, somewhat important, not very important, not important at all, or would it be important to you but you can't or have no choice because they don't offer Orthodox services."

    Resident responds, "It's important for me to go to Orthodox services if they were offered, but they aren't. So, can't do or no choice."

    Coding: F0500I would be **coded 5, important, but can't do or no choice.**

2. Resident answers, "My pastor sends taped services to me that I listen to in my room on Sundays. I don't participate in the services here."

> **DEFINITIONS:**
>
> **PARTICIPATE IN RELIGIOUS SERVICES**
> Any means of taking part in religious services or practices, such as listening to services on the radio or television, attending services in the facility or in the community, or private prayer or religious study.
>
> **RELIGIOUS PRACTICES**
> Rituals associated with various religious traditions or faiths, such as washing rituals in preparation for prayer, following kosher dietary laws, honoring holidays and religious festivals, and participating in communion or confession.

Interviewer probes, "You said your pastor sends you taped services. Would you say that it is very important, somewhat important, not very important, or not important at all, to you that you are able to listen to those tapes from your pastor?"

Resident responds, "Oh, that's very important."

Coding: F0500I would be **coded 1, very important**.

F0600: Daily and Activity Preferences Primary Respondent

Item Rationale

This item establishes the source of the information regarding the resident's preferences.

Coding Instructions

- **Code 1, resident**: if resident was the primary source for the preference questions in F0400 and F0500.

- **Code 2, family or significant other:** if a family member or significant other was the primary source of information for F0400 and F0500.
- **Code 9, interview could not be completed**: if F0400 and F0500 could not be completed by the resident, a family member, or a representative of the resident.

F0700: Should the Staff Assessment of Daily and Activity Preferences Be Conducted?

Item Rationale

Health-related Quality of Life

- Resident interview is preferred as it most accurately reflects what the resident views as important. However, a small percentage of residents are unable or unwilling to complete the interview for Daily and Activity Preferences.
- Persons unable to complete the preference interview should still have preferences evaluated and considered.

Planning for Care

- Even though the resident was unable to complete the interview, important insights may be gained from the responses that were obtained, observing behaviors, and observing the resident's affect during the interview.

Steps for Assessment

1. Review resident, family, or significant other responses to F0400A-H and F0500A-H.

Coding Instructions

- **Code 0, no:** if Interview for Daily and Activity Preferences items (F0400 and F0500) was completed by resident, family, or significant other. Skip to Section G, Functional Status.
- **Code 1, yes:** if Interview for Daily and Activity Preferences items (F0400 through F0500) were not completed because the resident, family, or significant other was unable to answer 3 or more items (i.e. 3 or more items in F0400 through F0500 were coded as 9 or "-").

Coding Tips and Special Populations

- If the total number of unanswered questions in F0400 through F0500 is equal to 3 or more, the interview is considered incomplete.

F0800: Staff Assessment of Daily and Activity Preferences

Item Rationale

Health-related Quality of Life

- Alternate means of assessing daily preferences must be used for residents who cannot communicate. This ensures that information about their preferences is not overlooked.

- Activities allow residents to establish meaning in their lives. A lack of meaningful and enjoyable activities can result in boredom, depression, and behavioral symptoms.

Planning for Care

- Caregiving staff should use observations of resident behaviors to understand resident likes and dislikes in cases where the resident, family, or significant other cannot report the resident's preferences. This allows care plans to be individualized to each resident.

Steps for Assessment

1. Observe the resident when the care, routines, and activities specified in these items are made available to the resident.
2. Observations should be made by staff across all shifts and departments and others with close contact with the resident.
3. If the resident appears happy or content (e.g., is involved, pays attention, smiles) during an activity listed in Staff Assessment of Daily and Activity Preferences item (F0800), then that item should be checked.

   If the resident seems to resist or withdraw when these are made available, then do not check that item.

Coding Instructions

Check all that apply in the last 7 days based on staff observation of resident preferences.

- **F0800A**. Choosing clothes to wear
- **F0800B**. Caring for personal belongings
- **F0800C**. Receiving tub bath
- **F0800D**. Receiving shower
- **F0800E**. Receiving bed bath
- **F0800F**. Receiving sponge bath
- **F0800G**. Snacks between meals
- **F0800H**. Staying up past 8:00 PM
- **F0800I**. Family or significant other involvement in care discussions
- **F0800J**. Use of phone in private
- **F0800K**. Place to lock personal belongings
- **F0800L**. Reading books, newspapers, or magazines
- **F0800M**. Listening to music
- **F0800N**. Being around animals such as pets
- **F0800O**. Keeping up with the news
- **F0800P**. Doing things with groups of people
- **F0800Q**. Participating in favorite activities
- **F0800R**. Spending time away from the nursing home
- **F0800S**. Spending time outdoors
- **F0800T**. Participating in religious activities or practices
- **F0800Z**. None of the above

G. Certification of Accuracy of MDS

The RAI is best accomplished by an IDT that includes health care professionals who have clinical knowledge about the resident, including the activity professional. All health professionals contributing to the assessment must sign their full signature with professional title and date and indicate the section of the MDS that they completed in Item X0400. Each person that completes information on the MDS is responsible for the accuracy of the items that they completed.

CFR Section 483.20(i) Interpretive Guidelines

Whether the MDS assessments are manually completed, or computer generated following data entry, each individual assessor is responsible for certifying the accuracy of responses relative to the resident's condition and discharge or entry status. Manually completed forms are signed and dated by each individual assessor the day they complete their portion(s) of the MDS record. When MDS forms are completed directly on the facility's computer (e.g., no paper form has been manually completed), then each individual assessor signs and dates a computer generated hard copy, or provides an electronic signature, after they review it for accuracy of the portion(s) they completed. Backdating completion dates is not acceptable — note that recording the actual date of completion is not considered backdating. For example, if an MDS was completed electronically and a hard copy was printed two days later, writing the date the MDS was completed on the hard copy is not considered backdating.

CMS's RAI Version 3.0 Manual Section Z0400
Signatures of Persons Completing the Assessment

Item Rationale

- *To obtain the signature of all persons who completed any part of the MDS. Legally, it is an attestation of accuracy with the primary responsibility for its accuracy with the person selecting the MDS item response. Each person completing a section or portion of a section of the MDS is required to sign the Attestation Statement.*

- *The importance of accurately completing and submitting the MDS cannot be over-emphasized.*

The MDS is the basis for the development of:

  — *an individualized care plan;*

  — *the Medicare Prospective Payment System*

  — *Medicaid reimbursement programs*

  — *quality monitoring activities, such as the quality indicator/quality measure*

> *reports*
>
> — *the data-driven survey and certification process*
>
> — *the quality measures used for public reporting*
>
> — *research and policy development.*

All staff who completed any part of the MDS must enter their signatures, titles, sections or portion(s) of section(s) they completed, and the date completed. If a staff member cannot sign Z0400 on the same day that he or she completed a section or portion of a section, when the staff member signs, use the date the item originally was completed.

Two or more staff members can complete items within the same section of the MDS. When filling in the information for Z0400, any staff member who has completed a subset of items within a section should identify which item(s) he/she completed within that section.

Nursing homes may use electronic signatures for medical record documentation, including the MDS, when permitted to do so by state and local law and when authorized by the nursing home's policy. Nursing homes must have written policies in place that meet any and all state and federal privacy and security requirements to ensure proper security measures to protect the use of an electronic signature by anyone other than the person to whom the electronic signature belongs. Although the use of electronic signatures for the MDS does not require that the entire record be maintained electronically, most facilities have the option to maintain a resident's record by computer rather than hard copy.

Surveyors will look at clinical records to make sure that the appropriate certifications are in place, including the certification of individual assessors of the accuracy and completion of the portion(s) of the assessment tracking form or face sheet that they completed. Section Z0400 (a) to (l) contains signatures of persons completing portions of the MDS or tracking forms. Section Z0400 also contains the certification statement that staff members must sign and date attesting to the accuracy of the portions of the MDS completed by each member of the IDT. The signature and date of the person completing a section of the MDS must reflect that date that the documentation was completed.

Read the Attestation Statement carefully. The activity professional's signature certifies that the information entered on the MDS, to the best of your knowledge, most accurately reflects the resident's status. Penalties may be applied for submitting false information.

The certification statement is as follows:

> *I certify that the accompanying information accurately reflects resident assessment information for this resident and that I collected or coordinated collection of this information on the dates specified. To the best of my knowledge, this information was collected in accordance with applicable Medicare and Medicaid requirements. I understand that this information is used as a basis for ensuring that residents receive appropriate and quality care, and as a basis for payment from federal funds. I further understand that payment of such federal funds and*

continued participation in the government-funded health care programs is conditioned on the accuracy and truthfulness of this information, and that I may be personally subject to or may subject my organization to substantial criminal, civil, and/or administrative penalties for submitting false information. I also certify that I am authorized to submit this information by this facility on its behalf.

MDS information is used for multiple purposes that rely on accurate information. First of all, the MDS is used for the development of the resident care plan. Additionally, the MDS is used to determine the amount of payment for Medicare Part A Prospective Payment System and for Medicaid payment in some states. Quality monitoring by CMS uses MDS data to calculate quality indicators used in the state survey process and quality measures that are posted on CMS's Internet Website Nursing Home Compare. Each professional contributing to the MDS must complete the MDS accurately to assure the integrity of these programs.

Interpretive Guidelines Section 483.20(j) Penalty for Falsification

... A pattern within a nursing home of clinical documentation or of MDS assessment or reporting practices that result in higher RUG scores, untriggering CAA(s), or unflagging QI(s), where the information does not accurately reflect the resident's status, may be indicative of payment fraud or avoidance of the quality monitoring process.

---

6. CARE AREA ASSESSMENTS

```
KEY POINTS AND SUMMARY OF CHAPTER

Activity pursuits are a need for all residents, not just those triggered by the MDS.

Data from the MDS is interpreted and combined with input from the interdisciplinary
team to develop a care plan that reflects the resident's unique needs, problems, or
strengths.

Working the Care Area Trigger (CAT) and writing a Care Area Assessment (CAA) is a
supplemental assessment process that links the MDS data to care planning.

Documentation of decision-making based on working the CAA is essential for the
development of a resident-centered care plan.
```

A. Using Care Area Assessment

CMS developed the Care Area Assessments (CAAs) to facilitate care planning from the information collected on the MDS and areas it triggered as needing additional assessment. Working the CAA is an essential process to develop a resident-specific care plan. Care Area Assessments guide staff to identify underlying causes and unique risk factors that may be reversed or to prevent further deterioration.

There are twenty areas addressed in the Care Area Assessments. One of the areas is Activities. However, activity professionals will find that other CAAs, such as cognition, communication, mood, and behavior, include information that influences the quality of the resident's life and activity choices. Care Area Triggers (CATS) are identified based on data entered on the MDS. The CATs are used to identify resident-specific problems, strengths, and preferences and provide a decision-making process for care plan development. The IDT with the input of the resident, family, or resident's representation determines when a problem or potential problem needs to be addressed in the care plan.

The CAAs are not done with quarterly or Medicare MDS. CAAs are only completed with comprehensive assessments, such as admission, annual, and significant change of condition. On a comprehensive assessment if a resident triggers the same CAA that triggered on the last comprehensive assessment, the CAA should be reviewed again. Even if the CAA is triggered for the same reason (no difference in MDS responses), there may be a new or changed related event identified during the CAA review that might call for a revision to the resident's care plan.

From CMS's RAI Version 3.0 Manual

The information in the MDS constitutes the core of the required State-specified Resident Assessment Instrument (RAI). Based on assessing the resident, the MDS identifies actual or potential areas of concern. The remainder of the RAI process supports the efforts of nursing home staff, health professionals, and practitioners to further assess these trigger areas of concern in order to identify, to the extent possible, whether the findings represent a problem or risk requiring further intervention, as well as the causes and risk factors related to the triggered care area under assessment. These conclusions then provide the basis for developing an individualized care plan for each resident.

The CAA process framework. The CAA process provides a framework for guiding the review of triggered areas, and clarification of a resident's functional status and related causes of impairments. It also provides a basis for additional assessment of potential issues, including related risk factors. The assessment of the causes and contributing factors gives the interdisciplinary team (IDT) additional information to help them develop a comprehensive plan of care.

When implemented properly, the CAA process should help staff:

- *Consider each resident as a whole, with unique characteristics and strengths that affect his or her capacity to function;*

- *Identify areas of concern that may warrant interventions;*

- *Develop, to the extent possible, interventions to help improve, stabilize, or prevent decline in physical, functional, and psychosocial well-being, in the context of the resident's condition, choices, and preferences for interventions; and*

- *Address the need and desire for other important considerations, such as advanced care planning and palliative care; e.g., symptom relief and pain management.*

The Care Area Assessment documents the rationale or the "thinking" to proceed or not proceed with care planning. Thoughtful CAAs will help staff identify ways to improve the outcome of care and ultimately the quality of life of residents in the nursing facility.

For example, a resident may be hard of hearing and the communications CAA is triggered. Risk factors and complications that would affect the resident's quality of life and activity participation should be addressed. The interdisciplinary team assesses the causal factors to determine if any are reversible or how the hearing deficit will be managed. The activity professional uses the review of the CAA to develop an activity care plan that meets this resident's specific and unique needs related to the hearing deficit.

When marking certain items on the MDS form, resident problems, needs, or strengths will be triggered. Care Area Triggers (CATs) identify potential problems that may possibly be reversed or improved. Triggers are a method to flag conditions that need further care area assessment.

While completing Section F of the MDS, the activity professional should be aware of data items that will trigger a CAT. Data in Section F triggers both the Activity CAT and the Psychosocial CAT. Data entered possibly by a different health care profession in Section D will also trigger the Activity CAT. CAT logic tables identify the triggering conditions for each CAT.

From CMS's RAI Version 3.0 Manual

10. Activities

The capabilities of residents vary, especially as abilities and expectations change, illness intervenes, opportunities become less frequent, and/or extended social relationships become less common. The purpose of the activities CAA is to identify strategies to help residents become more involved in relevant activities, including those that have interested and stimulated them in the past and/or new or modified ones that are consistent with their current functional and cognitive capabilities.

When this CAA is triggered, nursing home staff should follow their facility's chosen protocol or policy for performing the CAA. This CAA is triggered when the resident may have evidence of decreased involvement in social activities.

Activities CAT Logic Table

Triggering Conditions (any of the following):

1. *Resident has little interest or pleasure in doing things as indicated by:*

   D0200A1 = 1

2. *Staff assessment of resident mood suggests resident states little interest or pleasure in doing things as indicated by:*

   D0500A1 = 1

3. *Any 6 items for interview for activity preferences has the value of 4 (not important at all) or 5 (important, but cannot do or no choice) as indicated by:*

   Any 6 of F0500A through F0500H = 4 or 5

4. *Any 6 items for staff assessment of activity preference item L through T are not checked as indicated by:*

The information gleaned from the assessment should be used to identify residents who have either withdrawn from recreational activities or who are uneasy entering into activities and social relationships, to identify the resident's interests, and to identify any related possible contributing and/or risk factors. The next step is to develop an individualized care plan based directly on these conclusions. The care plan should focus on addressing the underlying cause(s) of activity limitations and the development or inclusion of activity programs tailored to the resident's interests and to his or her cognitive, physical/functional, and social abilities and improve quality of life.

The first two triggers rely on input to Section D Mood, which may be completed by another healthcare professional. In this case, the information on the MDS states that the resident has little interest or pleasure in doing things based on resident interview or staff assessment. This is important information for the activity professional for a resident-centered care plan. This data is not included in the trigger for any other CAA and is significant for activity care planning. Coordination with the IDT will assist in CAAs that address the potential problem actually triggered by the CAT.

The third trigger regarding activity preferences is based on resident interview. There are eight questions in Section F Item F0500 regarding the importance of activities to the resident while the resident is in the facility. The questions ask, "While you are in this facility, how important is it to you to":

    a. Have books, newspapers, and magazines to read

    b. Listen to music you like

    c. Be around animals such as pets

    d. Keep up with the news

    e. Do things with groups of people

    f. Do your favorite activities

    g. Go outside to get fresh air when the weather is good

    h. Participate in religious services or practices

The Activity CAT will trigger if any six of these eight items in F0500A through F0500H are scored with a value of "4" not important at all or a value of "5" important, but cannot do or no choice.

The fourth trigger regarding activity preferences is based on staff assessment of a resident who could not be interviewed. Item F0800 Staff Assessment of Daily and Activity Preferences is not done if there was an interview regarding daily and activity preferences in Items F0400-F0500. There are nine questions regarding the staff assessment of the resident. The areas are in Items F0800L through F0800T and assess whether the "Resident prefers":

    l. Reading books, newspapers, or magazines

---

m. Listening to music

n. Being around animals such as pets

o. Keeping up with the news

p. Doing things with groups of people

q. Participating in favorite activities

r. Spending time away from the nursing home

s. Spending time outdoors

t. Participating in religious activities

The Activity CAT will be triggered if any six out of the nine items in F0800L through F0800T are not checked.

Additionally, the activity professional should be aware that data entered in Section F will trigger the Psychosocial Well-Being CAT. Another health care professional may be responsible for working the CAA for Psychosocial. The need for interdisciplinary team participation is essential for the RAI process.

Psychosocial Well-Being CAT Logic Table

Triggering Conditions (listing of only those triggered by Section F)
3. Interview for activity preference item "How important is it to you to do your favorite activities?" has a value of 3 or 4 as indicated by:

   F0500F = 3 OR **F0500F** = 4

4. Staff assessment of daily and activity preferences did not indicate that resident prefers participating in favorite activities:

   F0800Q = not checked.

C. Documentation of the CAA Review

The CAA review process assists the activity professional to collect and analyze additional relevant information regarding the triggered condition. The purpose is to identify causal factors that affect the resident's condition and how factors contributing to the resident's problems can be eliminated or minimized.

1. Content of CAA Documentation

The CATs triggered by the MDS data identify suggested problems, needs, or strengths of the resident. For each CAT triggered, a decision is made whether or not to proceed to care planning. The decision-making process documents the causes and relationships between the resident's problems and is a method used to understand the

---

resident's needs. The care area assessment process includes documentation of the information that has been considered in the development of the care plan.

CAA documentation explains the rationale for care planning by describing how the IDT determined the underlying causes, contributing factors, and risk factors. Relevant documentation for each triggered CAA should describe:

- Causes and contributing factors;
- What exactly is the issue/problem for this resident and why it is a problem;
- Other triggered areas that affect or complicate the resident's needs;
- Risk factors related that affect the resident's function or quality of life;
- The need for additional evaluation by the attending physician or other health professionals; and
- The decision to care plan or not to care plan.

The activity professional determines whether a new care plan is needed or whether changes will be made in the resident's existing care plan. In order to provide continuity of care for the resident and effective communication to all persons involved in the resident's care, it is important that information from the assessment that led the team to their care planning decision be clearly documented.

Documentation about the resident's condition should support clinical decision-making regarding whether or not to proceed with a care plan for a triggered condition and the type(s) of care plan interventions that are appropriate for a particular resident.

2. Locations of CAA Documentation

Documentation of the CAA review process may appear anywhere in the clinical record according to facility policy. In most cases, the facility will have flexibility in documenting CAAs. CAA documentation is a written account of the team's clinical thought processes about the resident assessment findings.

Select the method or combination of methods that best fits with existing facility documentation practices. Some appropriate locations are

- CAA Resource Tool,
- narrative CAA summary,
- supplemental assessment forms, and
- other appropriately identified progress notes.

CMS's RAI MDS 3.0 Manual has provided CAA Resource Tools for each CAT. This information can be useful as a worksheet for a CAA Narrative Summary. To complete the CAA Resource Tool, simply check off areas that apply and add a narrative that describes the nature of the problem, risks, and complications, care plan factors, referrals, and rationale for care planning in the column titled "Supporting Documentation." Complete the Resource Tool with conclusions that describe the problem identified, significant risk factors, factors to consider in care plan development, referrals, and the rationale for proceeding or not proceeding to care planning.

Another option for documenting the CAA decision-making is to identify existing documentation in the chart, such as progress notes. Depending on facility policy, this may be a less reliable method than other systematic options previously discussed. Problems arise in that there is no guarantee that all elements of the required CAA documentation have already been addressed in the record. Additionally, this can also be a time consuming task to identify these entries which, if not found, will require additional time spent in completing the documentation.

When identifying existing information already in the record, the location of information must be clearly identified with the date.

History and Physical 7/20/11

Nursing Admission Note 11/5/11

Activity Progress Note 2/16/12

Supplemental assessments such as the activity needs assessment will most likely contain the required documentation. When using supplemental assessment forms, clearly state the reason to proceed or not proceed to care planning.

Select a method of documenting the CAA process that fits with existing facility documentation procedures. The facility does not have to restrict itself to one method. A combination of methods may be used on the same chart. Use methods that are routinely a part of your facility's clinical records. Examples of supplemental assessment forms are found in this book in Chapter 2, Selecting Forms.

STEPS TO COMPLETING CAA

1. After completing the MDS, review any MDS items and responses in Section F, as well as other interrelated sections, to determine if the Activity CAT has been triggered.

2. Conduct a thorough assessment of the resident based on the data that triggered the CAT.

3. Review the Care Area Resource Tool for Activity.

4. Document how any contributing factors affect the activity needs of the resident and any symptoms, possible risks, and contributing factors.

5. Obtain and consider input from resident, family, and/or resident's representative regarding the activity plan.

6. Analyze the findings in the context of their relationship to the care area and standards of practice. This should include a review of indicators and supporting documentation, including symptoms and causal and contributing factors, related to this care area. Draw conclusions about the causal/contributing factors and effect(s) on the resident, and document these conclusions in the Analysis of Findings section.

7. Decide whether referral to other disciplines is warranted and document this decision.

   If using the Care Area Resource Tool for CAA documentation.

8. Check the box in the left column if the item is present for this resident. Some of this information will be on the MDS — some will not.

---

9. In the right column the facility can provide a summary of supporting documentation regarding the basis or reason for checking a particular item or items. This could include the location and date of that information, symptoms, possible causal and contributing factors(s) for item(s) checked.

10. Decide whether referral to other disciplines is warranted and document this decision.

11. In the Care Plan Considerations section, document whether a care plan for the triggered care area will be developed and the reason(s) why or why not.

12. Information in the Supporting Documentation column can be used to populate the Location and Date of CAA Information column in Section V, Item V0200A (CAA Results) — for example, See Delirium CAA 4/30/11, H&P date 4/18/11.

The checklist of care-area-specific resources provided in the CMS RAI MDS 3.0 Manual are neither mandated, prescriptive, nor all-inclusive. They are provided only as a service to facilities. They do not constitute or imply endorsement by CMS or HHS.

D. Examples of CAA Documentation

The documentation of the CAA process can make a difference. Careful assessment can assist health professionals to identify factors that can improve the quality of life of residents in a nursing facility. Time and again there is evidence that residents who would have fallen through the cracks were identified by the RAI process and poor outcomes of care were avoided.

As the RAI has become an integral part of care delivery, many examples of successful interventions have been attributed to the RAI process. The following examples are two cases with similar MDS data but different underlying causes.

> **Example 1:** A resident triggered delirium and cognitive deficit. The review of the CAA determined that this is an established case of Alzheimer's dementia. A care plan was developed to promote self-sufficiency in a safe environment to enhance the quality of the resident's life, including a meaningful activity program specific to the resident's cognitive level.

> **Example 2:** Another resident also triggered delirium and cognitive deficit. However, the CAA review determined that the resident has diabetes that is out of control and has poor vision. By identifying the underlying causes, action steps were taken to stabilize those conditions. When the resident's diabetes came under control and he was properly oriented to the facility, the factors that triggered delirium and cognitive deficit disappeared. Activity programs were directed to orientation of the resident to daily activities and schedules. The room was arranged and self-help aids were made available. By identifying the resident's underlying problems, his quality of life was improved.

These example CAA assessments led to two different care plans and two different outcomes. Consistent care area assessment enables the health care professional to identify treatable underlying causes. Outcomes of care improve as skills in assessment improve. Problem identification and care plans driven by the CAA guidelines will lead to enhanced quality of life for each resident.

E. Activity Program Related CATs

Resident's strengths and needs in one area interrelate with strengths and needs in other areas. In addition to the information contained in Section F, other sections of the Minimum Data Set (MDS) will contain useful data for the development of the activity plan. Participation in the interdisciplinary team planning conference is an important step to integrate the activity plan with the comprehensive resident care plan. The activity professional will find that CATs other than Activities will require activity interventions and that activity interventions will be coordinated as part of care plans developed by other professional health disciplines.

Care Area Trigger	Interrelated concerns that may affect activity plan
Delirium	Lack of frequent reorientation, reassurance, reminders to help make sense of things
Cognitive Loss/ Dementia	Participates better in small group programs (F0800P, observation, record)
Visual Function	Is resident's environment adapted to his or her unique needs, such as availability of large print books, high wattage reading lamp, night light, etc.?
Communication	Communication is more successful with some individuals than with others. Identify and build on the successful approaches (from record, interviews, observation) Limited opportunities for communication due to social isolation or need for communication devices (from record, interviews) Use of communication devices (from record, observation) such as, hearing aid, written communication, sign language, Braille, signs, gestures, sounds, communication board, electronic assistive devices
Psychosocial Well-being	Customary lifestyle (from resident, family staff interviews, and clinical record) (Section F) • Was lifestyle more satisfactory to the resident prior to admission to the nursing home? • Has facility care plan to date been as consistent as possible with resident's prior lifestyle, preferences, and routines (F0400, F0600, F0800)?

Care Area Trigger	Interrelated concerns that may affect activity plan
	Strengths to build upon (from resident, family, staff interviews, and clinical record): • Activities in which resident appears especially at ease interacting with others • Certain situations appeal to resident more than others, such as small groups or 1:1 interactions rather than large groups • Certain individuals who seem to bring out a more positive, optimistic side of the resident • Positive traits that distinguished the resident as an individual prior to his or her illness • Things that gave the resident a sense of satisfaction earlier in his or her life
Mood State	Personal loss Recent move into or within the nursing home (A1700) Recent change in relationships, such as illness or loss of a relative or friend Recent change in health perception, such as perception of being seriously ill or too ill to return home (Q0300-Q0600) Clinical or functional change that may affect the resident's dignity, such as new or worsening incontinence, communication difficulties, or decline
Behavior Symptoms	Frustration due to problem communicating discomfort or unmet needs Fear due to not recognizing the environment or misinterpreting the environment or actions of others Departure from normal routines Noisy, crowded area Dimly let area Sensory impairment, such as hearing or vision problems Restraints (P0100) Need for repositioning (M1200)
Pain	Limits day-to-day activities (J0500B) (social events, eating in dining room, etc.)

Review all areas triggered to determine any interrelationships with the resident's activity needs. Include these areas in the Care Area Assessment for Activities and add appropriate interventions to the care plan.

F. CAA Summary Form Section V

The CAA Summary Section V0200 can be thought of as a roadmap between the MDS and the care plan. The location of the documentation of decision-making is identified, such as the supplemental activity needs assessment.

Documentation on Section V0200 CAA Summary Form includes:

- The identification of the CAAs triggered by the data collection in the MDS,
- A determination of whether to proceed to care planning based on the information collected for each resident, and
- Location of CAA summary information that documents the decision-making process.

The CAA Summary form is the final step in the comprehensive MDS. Each CAA triggered by the MDS data is identified and a decision to proceed or not proceed to care planning is recorded on the CAA Summary form. This form identifies the problems that were triggered, the decision to care plan, and the location of the supplemental assessment information.

The CAA summary form is an index to those items triggered by the MDS. The CAA is reviewed for each problem triggered. From this review, a decision is made whether to proceed or not proceed to care planning. When a CAA is triggered, it simply means that additional assessment is required. It does not mean that a care plan must be developed for that particular condition.

All residents will have activity pursuit needs. However, not all residents will trigger the Activities CAA, even though activity pursuits are a universal need for residents in nursing facilities. Care plans may be written for problems that are not identified through the MDS triggering process.

Finally, the location of the supplemental activity assessment information is identified. The location is usually in the activity assessment completed on admission. The facility may have other procedures for CAA narrative documentation such as specific narrative summary, CAA resource tools, or elsewhere in the clinical record according to facility procedures. Be specific when identifying the location of supplemental assessment, including dates. Do not identify locations that do not contain assessment information. Do not duplicate or re-summarize information unnecessarily.

7. CARE PLANS

KEY POINTS AND SUMMARY OF CHAPTER

An activity care plan is resident-centered and is a universal need for all residents.

The care plan is based on the assessment information gathered throughout the RAI process.

The care plan identifies resident problems, unique characteristics, strengths, and needs, sets time-limited goals, and specifies interventions that have been assigned to specific caregivers.

A comprehensive care plan is a "communication tool" of the interdisciplinary team to coordinate resident care.

A. Comprehensive Care Plans

A comprehensive care plan is essential for delivery of quality care and achievement of positive outcomes of care. The clinical record system hinges on this document. When all resident needs are identified and realistic goals set, the implementation of the plan will lead to the desired outcomes and quality of life for the resident. Unmet needs or unidentified problems can result in a decline in the resident condition and undesired outcomes of care.

Using the information gathered during the assessment process, a comprehensive plan of care is written with input from the interdisciplinary team. An appropriate care plan results from an analysis of consistent, reliable information, such as the data compiled by the MDS and other supplemental assessments. The benefit of a comprehensive care plan is that all caregivers are following the same interventions directed toward achieving common goals.

From CMA's RAI Version 3.0 Manual

The comprehensive care plan is an interdisciplinary communication tool. It must include measurable objectives and time frames and must describe the services that are to be furnished to attain or maintain the resident's highest practicable physical, mental, and psychosocial well-being. The care plan must be reviewed and revised periodically, and the services provided or arranged must be consistent with each resident's written plan of care... (The) nursing home must ... use the results of the assessments to develop, review, and revise the resident's comprehensive plan of care.

Good assessment is the starting point for good clinical problem solving and decision-making and ultimately for the creation of a sound care plan. The CAAs provide a link between the MDS and care planning. The care plan should be revised on an ongoing basis to reflect changes in the resident and the care that the resident is receiving.

The care plan is driven not only by identified resident issue and/or conditions but also by a resident's unique characteristics, strengths, and needs. A care plan that is based on a thorough assessment, effective clinical decision-making, and is compatible with current standards of clinical practice can provide a strong basis for optimal approaches to quality of care and quality of life needs of individual residents. A well-developed and executed assessment and care plan:

- *Looks at each resident as a whole human being with unique characteristics and strengths;*

- *Views the resident in distinct functional areas for the purpose of gaining knowledge about the resident's functional status (MDS);*

- *Gives the IDT a common understanding of the resident;*

- *Re-groups the information gathered to identify possible issues and/or conditions that the resident may have (i.e., triggers);*

- *Provides additional clarity of potential issues and/or conditions by looking at possible causes and risks (CAA process);*

- *Develops and implements an interdisciplinary care plan based on the assessment information gathered throughout the RAI process, with necessary monitoring and follow-up;*

- *Provides information regarding how the causes and risks associated with issues and/or conditions can be addressed to provide for a resident's highest practicable level of well-being (care planning);*

- *Re-evaluates the resident's status at prescribed intervals (i.e., quarterly, annually, or if a significant change in status occurs) using the RAI and then modifies the individualized care plan as appropriate and necessary.*

The interdisciplinary team develops a care plan that considers the resident's whole condition by:

- Identifying resident problems, unique characteristics, strength and needs;
- Establishing goals;
- Setting time limits in which to attain goals;
- Developing interventions to reach goals; and
- Assigning staff responsibility.

All residents have a need for activity planning, whether or not triggered by the MDS (Minimum Data Set). An activity care plan is a universal need for all residents. A care plan must be more than a paperwork exercise. It is a proven tool for delivering and improving resident care.

By the very fact that residents are in a nursing facility, they can no longer satisfy their need for diversional or recreational activities. They cannot go out to lunch with friends, shopping, to a theater, or any other usual pursuits because of their physical requirements for hospitalization. It is the activity program's goals to identify residents' preferences and build on their strengths. Care plans are developed to supply meaningful diversions and stimulation within the facility environment.

B. Regulations for Comprehensive Care Plans

During the survey process, a sample of care plans will be reviewed. Surveyors will focus on the unique needs of each resident as identified in triggered CAAs, such as: cognitive deficit or intact, vision or hearing problems, communication or language barriers, and customary routines prior to admission. Section 483.20(k) of the federal regulations set the guidelines for evaluating compliance of comprehensive care plans.

Comprehensive Care Plans

CFR Section 483.10(d)(3) The resident has the right to — unless adjudged incompetent or otherwise found to be incapacitated under the laws of the State, participate in planning care and treatment or changes in care and treatment.

CFR Section 483.20(d) (A facility must...) use the results of the assessment to develop, review, and revise the resident's comprehensive plan of care.

CFR Section 483.20(k) Comprehensive Care Plans

(1) The facility must develop a comprehensive care plan for each resident that includes measurable objectives and timetables to meet a resident's medical, nursing, and mental and psychosocial needs that are identified in the comprehensive assessment.

The plan of care must describe the following:
    (i) The services that are to be furnished to attain or maintain the resident's highest practicable physical, mental, and psychosocial well-being...
    (ii) Any services that would otherwise be required ... but are not provided due to the resident's exercise of rights ... including the right to refuse treatment.

(2) A comprehensive care plan must be —
    (i) Developed within 7 days after the completion of the comprehensive assessment;
    (ii) Prepared by an interdisciplinary team, that includes the attending physician, a registered nurse with responsibility for the resident, and other appropriate

---

staff in disciplines as determined by the resident's needs, and, to the extent practicable, the participation of the resident, the resident's family, or the resident's legal representative; and

(iii)Periodically reviewed and revised by a team of qualified persons after each assessment.

Interpretive Guidelines: Section 483.20(k) Comprehensive Care Plans

An interdisciplinary team, in conjunction with the resident, resident's family, surrogate, or representative, as appropriate, should develop quantifiable objectives for the highest level of functioning the resident may be expected to attain, based on the comprehensive assessment. The interdisciplinary team should show evidence in the CAA summary or clinical record of the following:

- *The resident's status in triggered CAA areas;*

- *The facility's rationale for deciding whether to proceed with care planning; and*

- *That the facility considered the development of care planning interventions for all CAAs triggered by the MDS.*

The care plan must reflect intermediate steps for each outcome objective if identification of those steps will enhance the resident's ability to meet his/her objectives. Facility staff will use these objectives to monitor resident progress. Facilities may, for some residents, need to prioritize their care plan interventions. This should be noted in the clinical record or on the plan of care.

The requirements reflect the facility's responsibilities to provide necessary care and services to attain or maintain the highest practicable physical, mental, and psychosocial well-being, in accordance with the comprehensive assessment and plan of care. However, in some cases, a resident may wish to refuse certain services or treatments that professional staff believe may be indicated to assist the resident in reaching his or her highest practicable level of well-being. Desires of the resident should be documented in the clinical record.

The content of the care plan will be evaluated by surveyors to determine if the activity program is suitable for the individual resident.

For example:

- If a resident does not easily understand English, is it suitable for the resident to attend a News Talk program that is in English?
- If a resident has severely impaired vision, are radios or music part of their activity program?
- Is the activity program the appropriate level for enjoyment by a cognitively impaired resident?
- Are residents with short attention spans placed close to the activity program's action in an attempt to stimulate them?

Surveyors also will determine if the care plan is carried out as planned. For example, activity attendance records will be checked to determine if the resident has attended suitable activities at the frequency identified in the care plan goal statement. Resident's will be observed to determine how their leisure time is being spent. Specifically, surveyors will look at residents who spend long hours without any apparently meaningful activity. Are they simply sitting in the hallways without being involved in any apparent type of meaningful activity?

Should a care plan not work or goals not be met, the care plan needs to be adjusted and different approaches tried. For example, the activity care plan goals and interventions should be revised if the resident's attendance at group activity programs has decreased or the resident no longer participates actively or falls asleep during programs. To determine if a care plan is not working, review the care plan goals. If the goals are not being met, the approaches in the care plan should be reviewed and new approaches developed.

A reassessment of the resident that evaluates any underlying causal factors that may contribute to the lack of success of the care plan must be documented. Such reassessments may be completed quarterly during the regular review of MDS information or at anytime in between when it is identified that the goals of the care plan are not being met or there is a significant change in condition.

Survey Procedures and Probes
Section 483.20(k)(1) Comprehensive Care Plans

- *Does the care plan address the needs, strengths, and preferences identified in the comprehensive resident assessment?*

- *Is the care plan oriented toward preventing avoidable declines in functioning or functional levels?*

- *How does the care plan attempt to manage risk factors?*

- *Does the care plan build on resident strengths?*

- *Does the care plan reflect standards of current professional practice?*

- *Do treatment objectives have measurable outcomes?*

- *Corroborate information regarding the resident's goals and wishes for treatment in the plan of care by interviewing resident, especially those identified as refusing treatment.*

- *Determine whether the facility has provided adequate information to the resident so that the resident was able to make an informed choice regarding treatment.*

- *If the resident has refused treatment, does the care plan reflect the facility's efforts to find alternative means to address the problem?*

Residents have the right to refuse to participate in activity programs. However, the resident should be assessed to determine the reasons that the resident does not wish to participate. Alternate activities, such as in-room music and books, should be provided, as well as assessing family or other significant support that involves the resident with meaningful leisure time.

If the resident's refusal results in a significant change, the interdisciplinary team should reassess the resident and institute care-planning changes. For example, if a resident refuses to leave his or her room and exhibits symptoms of depression, the care plan could be revised with interventions, such as psychiatric consult and drug and non-drug interventions to manage depression.

C. Procedures for Care Planning

A plan is developed which outlines the care to be given, the objectives to be accomplished and the professional discipline responsible for each element of care. The care plan should be initiated on admission for any immediate needs. A comprehensive care plan is completed seven days following the completion of the resident assessment instrument (RAI).

A care plan is at the heart of daily care delivery and improving the quality of the resident's life in the facility. Using the information gathered by assessment, a care plan is a blueprint for meeting the needs of the resident.

Periodically, the resident care plan is reviewed, evaluated, and updated by the health professionals involved in the care of the resident. At a minimum the plan is reviewed quarterly by the interdisciplinary team and coordinated with each minimum data set (MDS) assessment. The care plan is revised more often if there is a change in the resident's condition or the goals of the care plan are not achieved.

PROCEDURE FOR WRITING CARE PLANS

1. On admission a resident care plan is started with all known immediate problems and needs for the resident. For the activities program input to the care, welcoming and orientation needs should be addressed.
2. A comprehensive care plan is developed for each resident that includes measurable objectives and timetables to meet a resident's medical, nursing, and mental and psychosocial needs that are identified through the comprehensive assessment process.
3. The resident's problems and needs are identified from those triggered by the Minimum Data Set, review of the physician's orders for services to be provided or withheld, and input from supplemental assessments of other appropriate staff in disciplines determined by the resident's needs. All residents need activity input to the care plan, even though the Activities CAA did not trigger. Activity plans are a universal need for all residents.
4. The Resident Care Plan includes input from all professionals involved in the care of the resident. Every effort should be made to give the resident, the resident's family, or the resident's legal representative an opportunity to contribute to the care plan.
5. Short-Term Goals (Objectives) are identified for each problem in measurable, observable terms. Goals provide a mechanism for evaluating resident progress.
6. A realistic time limit in which to accomplish each goal is established. If a problem is of an ongoing nature, indicate "q 3 months" as the time limit.

7. Care to be given (interventions) specify methods to be implemented to accomplish the objective for each problem.
8. The professional discipline responsible for each intervention is identified.
9. The professional entering the problem signs their initials and verifies the initials with the full signature.
10. As the resident's condition or capacity changes, the resident care plan is updated. The date indicates when a new problem was identified and care planned.
11. After each quarterly MDS assessment, the plan is reviewed, evaluated, and updated by all professional personnel involved in the care of the resident.
12. The date of each quarterly review is indicated on the resident care plan.
13. When a problem is resolved, a yellow highlighter pen is used to mark through the problem. The word "Resolved" and the date are recorded.
14. The care plan is written in ink or generated by computer. The care plan is a part of the resident's clinical record.

D. Problem Identification

Following the completion of the Resident Assessment Instrument (MDS) and the supplemental assessments, all information about the resident is reviewed. The MDS will trigger or identify certain problems that need to be addressed in the care plan. From the composite of all information known about each resident, problems and needs are identified. However, the MDS is a minimum data set and will not trigger all of the resident's problems and needs. These additional problems and needs will be identified by the interdisciplinary team through the supplemental assessment process. Remember that activities are a universal need for all residents in a nursing facility.

Writing the resident's needs on the care plan is an important first step. Style issues are secondary. The resident's needs can be listed as problem statements, CAA titles, nursing diagnoses, medical diagnoses or any other format that staff understands. When a need is identified, staff should be encouraged to write it down, regardless of the words used. Federal regulations do not contain a required format or mandated terminology.

Problems/needs statements have two components:

- First a description of the problem/need stated in functional or behavioral terms.
- Second is the underlying cause to identify the physical and/or mental limitations and/or strengths.

EXAMPLES OF PROBLEM STATEMENTS

Description of Problems, Strengths, or Needs	Underlying Cause (due to)(related to)
Complaints of boredom, loneliness	Removal from normal interpersonal and social contact
Constant demands and irritability	Refusal to accept limitations or participate in rehabilitation efforts
Decreased participation in activity programs	Visual impairment Hearing deficit Foreign language

Description of Problems, Strengths, or Needs	Underlying Cause (due to)(related to)
Decreased strength/mobility	Arthritis Pain Lack of motivation
Diversional activity deficit	Decreased stamina Loss of mobility Confusion and short attention span Inappropriate group behavior Refuses to participate in group activities
Lack of social interaction	Withdrawal from social contact Lack of motivation Refuses to participate in group activities
Limited interaction with others	Expressed preference for room activities
Needs in-room, bed appropriate activities	Non-weight-bearing status
Non-responsive to environment	Cerebral vascular accident
Short attention span and restlessness	Cognitive deficit Noise intolerance
Uncooperative/disruptive behavior	Mental confusion Inability to communicate needs
Withdrawal from social and interpersonal interactions	Recent loss of loved one Relocation to nursing facility

E. Setting Goals

Based on the resident assessment, long-term and short-term goals are developed. A long-term goal identifies the expected outcome for the resident's stay. Short-term goals identify the expected results of care provided. Goals are dynamic and may be changed frequently as the resident progresses or regresses.

1. Long-Term Goals

Long-term goals address the expected outcome of the hospitalization and are general in nature. Residents in nursing facilities have three general types of long-term goals:

- Rehabilitative goals that expect a resident to return to a previous level of functioning or a higher level of functioning.
- Maintenance goals that expect a resident to remain at the same level of functioning and not deteriorate.
- Supportive goals to keep the resident comfortable for those who are terminal or have a progressive disease process.

2. Short-Term (Intermediate) Goals

Each individual problem on the care plan should have a goal to address the immediate expectations to be achieved. Once a short-term goal is achieved, a new more ambitious goal can be developed if appropriate. The key to successful care planning is setting realistic, resident-oriented goals that are attainable for the resident.

Realistic goals answer the questions:

- Can the resident achieve the goal with his/her functional limitations?
- How will resident's strengths help achieve the goal?

Resident-oriented goals answer the questions:

- Does the resident want to achieve the goal?
- Is this outcome desired by the resident and family?

3. Goal Statements

Objectives or goals are written in measurable terms. A measurable goal is a phrase or statement by which the resident's progress can be evaluated in objective terms by any knowledgeable health care professional. A measurable goal specifies the amount of time and level of involvement of the resident in activities of his or her choice.

Subjective (Not Measurable): Resident will be less depressed.

Objective (Measurable): Resident will select three group activities to participate in each week (if the depression resulted in withdrawal from social contact).

Goals should include, whenever possible, resident strengths. Strengths may include: adequate vision, motivation for getting well, participation of family or friends.

Goals are an expression in objective and realistic measurements of the expected outcome of the planned interventions. The goal statements include:

- Specific activity or behavior is desired,
- A standard of objective measurement, and
- Time frame within which to accomplish the desired outcome of care.

The terminology for stating goals has three parts. First, identify what outcome is expected or desired. Next describe what measurement will determine if the resident has achieved the goals. And finally, how long it will take to reach the goals.

4. Time Limits

Time limits for goals may be documented in several ways.

- Included in the goal statement

  by (date)
  within two weeks
  for the next three months

- Included on the care plan form that has a column for

> time limit
> target date
> next review date

For example:

The resident will attend group activity programs without disruptive behavior (crying or calling out) for at least one half hour within 90 days (or specify a date).

It is recommended that time limits be set for no longer than three months. The time limit can then be updated during the quarterly review of the care plan.

EXAMPLES OF GOAL STATEMENTS

Desired outcomes	Demonstrated by (measurement)
The resident will respond to daily stimulation	By opening eyes
The resident will visit with volunteer _____ times per week	To assist with letter writing
The resident will attend group activity for fifteen minutes	Without disruptive behavior (wandering)
The resident will attend exercise class _____ times per week for fifteen minutes	Be able to catch beach ball and return throw
The resident will have at least ____ books at bedside and glasses within reach at all times	Be able to select books of interest from library cart
The resident will attend current events program daily	Be able to identify month and current season of year
The resident will sit in day room for at least one hour each afternoon	Respond verbally to conversation
The resident will attend exercise class daily	Will increase time of activity participation to 15 minutes daily
The resident will participate in morning and afternoon activity programs daily	Will be able to identify staff by name and recognize roommate/family and volunteer visitor
The resident will participate in bridge group/bible study and happy hour at least daily	Will actively lead groups
The resident will respond to sensory stimulation activities	Calm demeanor
The resident will be able to communicate needs	By use of communication board

FORMAT FOR GOAL STATEMENT

Desired behavior:	The resident will actively interact with care or activity staff at least five times per day during group activities, one-on-one sessions, and/or ADLs.
Measurable objective:	Responds to questions States name when asked Makes eye contact during activity Tracks ball with eyes Hits ball when directed toward staff Sings/mouths words to song Keeps time to music with rhythm instrument
Time limit for goal:	Date to be accomplished

F. Interventions

Once the expected outcome is agreed upon, the steps to be taken to achieve the goal are outlined. The discipline responsible for each step is specified.

Interventions or approaches answer the question of how to assist the resident to meet the care plan goals. Terminology should be appropriate and easily understood by the discipline that will be implementing the approach.

Interventions are the actions planned to assist the resident to achieve the desired goal or outcomes of care. They outline:

- The steps to be taken,
- Specific services to be offered, and
- Who is responsible.

1. Terminology for Interventions

The interventions or approaches are statements of actions and steps that will be done to help the resident in achieving the stated goal. Identify specific services to be offered.

A format for the approaches should be:

- Arrange attendance at (specify which activities)
- 1:1 visits (specify activity, e.g., conversation, tactile stimulation, sensory stimulation)
- Involve family/volunteer (how, e.g., take resident out of facility once a week, read correspondence to resident)

For example, an approach can be written as:

Activity Director will invite resident to attend Thursday afternoon music program. Resident will be asked to participate in selection of music.

Responsibility for the interventions can be documented in several ways:

- include in the approach/intervention a statement that
  - Activity Director will
  - by social worker
  - by certified nursing assistant
- include in the care plan form a column to identify
  - responsible discipline

EXAMPLES OF INTERVENTIONS

Actions to be taken	Specific services
Attend arts and crafts weekly	Remind resident to finish project
Escort to morning exercise	Praise resident for effort
Active participation	In resident council
Attend happy hour	Offer snacks and nourishment
Volunteer visit weekly	Take outside to garden Assist in tending potted plants
Provide careful supervision during craft classes	Be alert that resident may place items in mouth
Family visit every evening	To assist with feeding dinner
Engage resident in conversation	Call resident by first name
Provide training on communication board	For basic ADL needs
Counsel resident regarding angry outbursts	Encourage discussion of feelings
Counsel resident regarding inappropriate language	Praise resident for efforts
Arrange attendance at dieter's support group	Encourage verbal participation
No morning activity participation	Allow resident to sleep in
Provide small watering can	For tending indoor plants in room
Place in front row for movies	Be sure that hearing aid is working and resident is wearing glasses

G. Care Plan Conference

The care plan is based upon the information collected in the Minimum Data Set as well as information gathered by the interdisciplinary care team. The plan is started at the time of admission for the resident's immediate needs. The comprehensive care plan is developed by the interdisciplinary team within seven days of completion of the Resident Assessment Instrument.

At a minimum the interdisciplinary team should include the licensed nurse responsible for the resident, the certified nursing assistant assigned to the resident, the activity director, social worker, and dietitian or dietary manager. If the resident is receiving restorative therapy, the therapists should attend.

Although it is not required that an attending physician attend the interdisciplinary team conference, the physician should review the care plan to assure that it is appropriate for the resident. This may be indicated by signing approval on the care plan or by writing an order that the care plan has been reviewed and approved.

To assure that the activity plan is not in conflict with the physician's treatment plan, it is good practice to request physician orders for:

1. use of alcoholic beverage,
2. deviations from therapeutic diet,
3. permission to leave facility for outing, and/or
4. ability to participate in physical exercise programs.

When setting goals, resident and family cooperation and understanding is needed so all may work toward a common end. Participation by the resident or resident's family/legal representative is essential for the success of care planning. The care plan should be resident-oriented and include opportunities for the resident to exercise choice and self-determination, whenever possible. Do not underestimate the potential for success and positive outcomes that result from resident and family involvement in care planning.

Interpretive Guidelines §483.20(k)(2) Interdisciplinary Team

As used in this requirement, "Interdisciplinary" means that professional disciplines, as appropriate, will work together to provide the greatest benefit to the resident. It does not mean that every goal must have an interdisciplinary approach. The mechanics of how the interdisciplinary team meets its responsibilities in developing an interdisciplinary care plan (e.g., a face-to-face meeting, teleconference, written communication) is at the discretion of the facility.

The physician must participate as part of the interdisciplinary team, and may arrange with the facility for alternative methods, other than attendance at care planning conferences, of providing his/her input, such as one-on-one discussions and conference calls.

... The facility has a responsibility to assist residents to participate, e.g., helping residents, and families, legal surrogates, or representatives understand the assessment and care planning process; when feasible, holding care planning meetings at the time of day when a resident is functioning best; planning enough time for information exchange

---

and decision making; encouraging a resident's advocate to attend (e.g. family member, friend) if desired by a resident.

The resident has the right to refuse specific treatments and to select among treatment options before the care plan is instituted. The facility should encourage residents, legal surrogates, and representatives to participate in care planning, including attending care planning conferences if they so desire.

While Federal regulations affirm the resident's right to participate in care planning and to refuse treatment, the regulations do not create the right for a resident, legal surrogate, or representative to demand that the facility use specific medical intervention or treatment that the facility deems inappropriate. Statutory requirements hold the facility ultimately accountable for the resident's care and safety, including clinical decisions.

Probes §483.20(k)(2):

- *Was interdisciplinary expertise utilized to develop a plan to improve the resident's functional abilities?*

- *Is there evidence of physician involvement in development of the care plan (e.g., presence at care plan meetings, conversations with team members concerning the care plan, conference calls)?*

- *In what ways do staff involve residents and families, surrogates, and/or representatives in care planning?*

- *Do staff make an effort to schedule care plan meetings at the best time of the day for residents and their families?*

- *Do facility staff attempt to make the process understandable to the resident/family?*

- *Ask residents whether they have brought questions or concerns about their care to the attention of facility's staff. If so, what happened as a result?*

H. Interdisciplinary Care Plan

Coordinated team planning is essential for meeting all of the resident needs and achieving good outcomes. The activity professional has the lead responsibility in the development of the activity plan based on the Activities CAA. It is also appropriate for the activity professional to provide input and accept responsibility in several other CAA areas.

The care plan complex consists of the problem statement, the goals, and the approaches. In some facilities, each discipline writes its own problem complex. However, more than one discipline may need to provide input regarding the same problem. An interdisciplinary problem complex includes input from all appropriate disciplines to the problem statement, the goals, and the approaches. More than one discipline may be identified as responsible for implementing the plan.

The interdisciplinary team may find during their discussions that several problem conditions have a related cause but appear as one problem for the resident. Or they may find that they stand alone and are unique. Goals and approaches for each problem condition may be overlapping, and consequently the interdisciplinary team may decide to address the problem conditions in combination on the care plan.

CMS's RAI Version 3.0 Manual

A separate care plan is not necessarily required for each area that triggers a CAA. Since a single trigger can have multiple causes and contributing factors and multiple items can have a common cause or related risk factors, it is acceptable and may sometimes be more appropriate to address multiple issues within a single care plan segment or to cross-reference related interventions from several care plan segments.

Interdisciplinary input can be accomplished in two ways:

- Each discipline has a clearly identified problem complex written in each care plan.
- Each discipline contributes causal factors to the problem statements, goals unique to their discipline, and approaches they plan to implement or recommend. Each discipline would initial the input to the various problem complexes to which they contributed.

For example, the activity professional will provide input and include activity plan approaches for problems identified by several of the CAAs.

Delirium
Delirium is a symptom of a variety of acute, treatable illnesses. Even with successful treatment of cause(s) and associated symptoms, it may take several weeks before cognitive abilities return to pre-delirium status.

Problem and Goal Statement	Interventions (by Activities)
Delirium As evidenced by 　Disorderly thinking Related to 　Recent surgery 　Pain medication Goal: Will be oriented to time, place, and person by two weeks Pain level will be reduced to mild pain daily by day 5	Ensure access to clock and calendar in room One-to-one visits twice a day to reorient to time, place, and person Bring to music programs 3 times a week Ask family to bring radio or CD player for in room soft music

Cognitive Loss/Dementia

The cognitive loss/dementia CAA focuses on declining or worsening cognitive abilities that threaten a person's independence and increase the risk for long-term nursing home placement or impair the potential for return to the community.

Problem and Goal Statement	Interventions (by Activities)

Cognitive Decline
As evidenced by
    Short-term memory loss
Related to
    Alzheimer's disease
 	
Goal:
Will actively participate in two activities of choice daily
Will make choices between two options
	Assist with selection of menu items giving resident choices between two items
	
	Activities of interest are
	    Painting class
	    Sing-along
	    Excursions out of facility once a week
	    Pet visit by volunteers
	
	Active participation shown by
	    Appropriate verbalization
	    Appropriate interaction with activity materials

Visual Function

The quality of life can be improved for residents who have impaired vision through the use of appropriate visual appliances.

The consequences of vision loss are wide-ranging and can seriously affect physical safety, self-image, and participation in social, personal, self-care, and rehabilitation activities.

Problem and Goal Statement	Interventions (by Activities)

Impaired vision
As evidenced by
    Unable to read but can see large images
    Can see adequately for safe ambulation
Related to
    Macular degeneration, progressive
 	
Goal:
Will not injure self or others when ambulating
Will verbalize fears regarding sight
	Adapt environment to maximize visual functions
	    Large print signs
	    Large numbered phone
	    Night light
	
	Volunteer to read romance novels to resident three times a week
	
	Attend activities twice a day for current events, movies, music
	
	Escort to activity locations

Communications

Good communication enables residents to express emotion, listen to others, and share information. It also eases adjustment to a strange environment and lessens social isolation and depression.

As language use recedes with dementia, both the staff and the resident must expand their nonverbal communication skills — one of the most basic and automatic of human abilities. Touch, facial expression, eye contact, tone of voice, and posture all are powerful means of communicating with the demented resident, and recognizing and using all practical means is the key to effective communication.

Details of resident strengths and weaknesses in understanding, hearing, and expression are the direct or indirect focus of any treatment program.

For chronic conditions that are unlikely to improve, consider communication treatments or interventions that might compensate for losses (e.g., for moderately impaired residents with Alzheimer's, the use of short, direct phrases and tactile approaches to communication can be effective).

Problem and Goal Statement	Interventions (by Activities)

Communication impaired
As evidenced by
    Difficulty in understanding
    conversations
Related to
    Hard of hearing
    Speaks limited English, foreign
    language primary (Spanish)
 	
Goal:
Will understand simple sentences in
English
	Speak in short simple phrases
	
	Address resident from the left side which is the good ear
	
	Have family or interpreter available for medical care discussions
	
	Interact in non-verbal activities twice a day
	    Music
	    Painting
	    Pets

Psychosocial Well-Being

Well-being problems or needs to maintain psychosocial strengths are suggested if there is withdrawal from activities of interest or if the daily routine is very different from the prior pattern in the community.

Residents can withdraw or become distressed because they feel life lacks meaning. Activity programs are the main opportunity in nursing facilities for residents to socialize and find meaning in life.

Problem and Goal Statement	Interventions (by Activities)

Adjustment to facility
As evidenced by
    Expresses uneasiness about staying in
    the facility and expresses wish to go
    home
Related to
    Recent admission
 	
Goal:
Will participate in one daily activity of
choice for first month
Will verbalize positively to roommate
within next 7 days
	Refer to social worker for possible
	discharge planning
	
	Make sure activity calendar is available and
	invite to activity program every day
	
	If does not attend a program, follow up
	with one-to-one visit to determine if special
	interests can be accommodated
	
	Provide TV schedule for sports events

Mood State

Considered a problem when there is withdrawal from activities and/or reduced social interaction.

The passive resident with distressed mood may be overlooked. Such a resident may be erroneously assumed to have no mood state problem.

Problem and Goal Statement	Interventions (by Activities)

Mood decline
As evidenced by
    Insomnia
Related to
    Depression
 	
Goal:
Sleep 6-8 hours each night
	Provide PM snack of warm milk after
	resident has prepared for bed
	
	Participation in evening activity program at
	least 3 times a week

Behavior

Care plan development for residents who exhibit the behavioral symptoms of wandering, being verbally abusive, being physically aggressive, and/or exhibiting socially inappropriate behavioral symptoms.

Some resident may not be capable of meaningful communication. However, many of the seemingly incomprehensible behaviors (e.g., screaming, aggressive behavior) in which these individuals engage may constitute their only form of communication. By observing the behavior and the pattern of its occurrence, one can frequently come to some understanding of the needs of individuals. For example, residents who are restrained for their own safety may become noisy due to bladder or bowel urgency.

Use non-verbal communication techniques (e.g., touch, gesture) to encourage resident to respond.

Problem and Goal Statement	Interventions (by Activities)

Behavioral symptoms
As manifested by
    Wandering and attempting to leave the
    facility
Related to
    Alzheimer's dementia
 	
Goal:
Will be engaged in activities or with care staff during most likely times for wandering
Will not injure self or leave the facility without supervisions
	Make sure resident attends afternoon activity program since this is the time she is most restless
	
	Include in activities that are physically active such as exercise group
	
	One-to-one volunteer will take resident out on patio and walks in garden
	
	Include resident in excursion outside of the facility

Nutritional Status

Residents with loss of appetite may be helped by programs involving food preparation and that include refreshments.

Residents who are fearful, who pace or wander, withdraw from activities, cannot communicate, or refuse to communicate, often refuse to eat or will eat only a limited variety and amount of foods.

Problem and Goal Statement	Interventions (by Activities)

Nutritional status altered
As manifested by
    Recent 5% weight loss
Related to
    Decreased appetite
 	
Goal:
Will maintain weight or gain back weight loss
	Involve in activities relating to food such as cooking class on Thursday
	
	Offer snack during programs such as popcorn, juices, and cookies
	
	Encourage family to bring in foods that the resident likes. Store appropriately at nursing station.

Restraints

Many interventions may be as effective as or even more effective than restraints in managing a resident's needs, safety risks, and problems.

Problem and Goal Statement	Interventions (by Activities)

<u>Needs Lap Cushion</u>
    To prevent resident from slipping out of wheelchair
Related to
    Weakness due to old CVA
 	
<u>Goal:</u>
Will be able to sit comfortably and safely in wheelchair during afternoons
No falls or injury from wheelchair
	Resident will be up every afternoon and attend activities he prefers such as
	    Art class
	    Music programs
	    Pets
	    Sports on television
	
	Reposition resident every 2 hours
	
	CNA to toilet resident prior to bringing to afternoon activity program

8. PROGRESS NOTES

KEY POINTS AND SUMMARY OF CHAPTER

Progress notes evaluate the resident's response and the results of the implementation of the care plan.

Progress notes should be written at least quarterly and more frequently if the resident has a significant change in condition.

Progress notes evaluate the outcome of the care plan. They are the final step of the documentation process. Good clinical progress notes communicate relevant and essential information in a concise manner. The resident's condition is described and response to interventions is observed in measurable terms. The activity professional must have the ability to identify clinically and/or legally significant events that require narrative documentation.

The purpose of progress notes is to:

- evaluate the resident's response to the plan of care and treatment.
- document the progress, maintenance, or regress in respect to the goals identified in the care plan.

When writing progress notes, the problems and needs of the resident that are identified in the care plan must be reviewed. The progress notes describe the resident's response to the interventions in the care plan. Any discrepancy between what is actually happening and what was planned needs to be clarified at this time. The assessment, the care plan, and the progress notes must agree in content.

A. Steps for Writing Progress Notes

Before writing a progress note follow these steps:

- Observe the resident's response to activity interventions.
- Discuss the resident with other professional staff to identify any changes in condition.
- Review physician orders for new or discontinued orders that may influence the resident's activity level.
- Review attendance records and flow sheets to identify subtle changes in resident behavior.

- Review previous progress notes to evaluate if the resident has changed or goals have not been met.
- Update the care plan if resident's activity level has changed.

B. Content of Progress Notes

Activity progress notes are written at least quarterly to evaluate the resident's progress, regress, or maintenance of the goals specified in the care plan. A progress note must be accurate, objective, and complete.

Descriptions should be specific to the resident's condition. Observe for objective findings. Describe what is seen. If the resident makes subjective statements, record them as "Resident states that ..."

Avoid terms that are nonspecific. For example, usually, frequently, at times, or occasionally are not measurable. Measurable documentation will state the number of times, how many times, what time something occurs.

The content of a progress note evaluates the goals identified in the care plan, response to interventions and treatments, and any new or short-term problems. Progress notes must be concise. Do not repeat a description of the care plan. Do not repeat information contained elsewhere in the health record unless there is more explanation needed.

Progress notes document the results of the care plan:

- How did the resident respond or adjust to the placement in the facility?
- How does the resident interact with staff and other residents?
- What is the resident doing now that he or she did not do in the past?
- Did an intervention not produce the anticipated result?
- What has been the degree of success or lack of success in attaining a specific goal?
- How has the resident changed since the care plan was written? Are there any new or short-term goals?
- What actions have been taken to resolve problems and how has the resident responded?
- Is the resident satisfied with the activity program?

C. Flow Sheets

Flow sheets are used to document resident information to be compared over a period of time. Flow sheets may be used to document activity program interventions and level of participation. Such flow sheets with information pertinent to the activity program may include:

- Attendance records
- One-to-one visit logs

Flow sheets enable the activity professional to document and review data in a quick and efficient manner. Also when evaluating the resident's condition, data can be easily found and compared. Use flow sheets to track resident participation in activity programs over time. Attendance logs will indicate frequency of participation or identify trends such as refusing to attend certain activities.

Review all flow sheets to gather information prior to the quarterly interdisciplinary team conference and to assist in writing the quarterly activity progress note.

D. Timing of Progress Notes

Quarterly narrative notes are written by the activity program staff to evaluate in descriptive terms the progress or lack of progress toward the goals set in the care plan. Identify new problems as they occur and evaluate the resident's response to care and treatment.

Establish a schedule for writing quarterly progress notes. Spread the work over a period of time so each resident can be evaluated individually. It is most efficient to coordinate the writing of quarterly progress notes with the interdisciplinary team conference.

Be alerted to the quarterly update of the Minimum Data Set. Any significant change or deterioration in the resident's activities of daily living skills may change a resident's level of participation in the activity program.

Meaningful and informative progress notes shall also be written as often as the resident's condition warrants.

- If the resident's condition changes
- On readmission following a temporary discharge to evaluate any change in the resident's activity needs
- At any more frequent intervals as specified by state regulations

If a resident is readmitted to the facility from an acute hospital, the activity director must assess the resident's activity status at that time. Often level of participation will change, if only temporarily following hospitalization. The resident may have lost strength in the hospital due to the acute illness. There may be a new diagnosis, medications or treatments, or a change in functional level or mental acuity that will require an alteration of the activity plan.

E. Inappropriate Notes

Remember that the clinical record is the resident's record. Information contained in the record describes the resident's condition, problems, needs, and treatment provided. Information regarding the facility's problems is not a part of the resident's treatment. Documentation in the clinical record reflects the professionalism of the person making the notes.

Do not write items in the record that are not related to the care of the resident. Complaints about other staff, blaming, or criticizing others are not appropriate in the clinical record. The mechanism for making such complaints should be done by an administrative memorandum.

When writing narrative notes:

- Use specific language. Avoid vague or generalized statements.

- Do not speculate; state only the facts and objective information.
- Describe symptoms by manifestation or behavior.
- Use quotation marks for statements made by resident.

If it is necessary to refer to another resident to describe an event, the other resident's name should not be used. The clinical record should contain only documentation that pertains to the direct care of the resident.

9. RESIDENT AND FAMILY COUNCIL

```
┌ ─ ─ ─ ─ ─ ─ ─ ─ ─ ─ ─ ─ ─ ─ ─ ─ ─ ─ ─ ─ ─ ─ ─ ─ ─ ┐
        KEY POINTS AND SUMMARY OF CHAPTER

  Resident and Family Councils provide an opportunity to improve quality of life in the
  facility and result in positive resident/family satisfaction.

  Surveyors interview residents and family members to determine if they are satisfied with
  care provided by the facility.

  Minutes and an action summary are documentation of the issues raised by the resident
  and family council and that the facility has made attempts to accommodate these
  recommendations
└ ─ ─ ─ ─ ─ ─ ─ ─ ─ ─ ─ ─ ─ ─ ─ ─ ─ ─ ─ ─ ─ ─ ─ ─ ─ ┘
```

The Resident and Family Councils provide an opportunity for choice and self-determination. By discussing and offering suggestions, the resident or family member can influence the quality of their life in the facility and resident and family satisfaction with the care provided.

Key steps in attaining resident and family satisfaction are

- participation in care planning,
- attendance at resident and family councils,
- ability to make choices, and
- mechanism to voice grievances.

A. Federal Regulations

Federal regulations provide for resident/family groups to discuss care and life in the facility and make recommendations. However, the regulations do not require that resident's organize a residents or family group. If no group exists, surveyors will determine if residents have attempted to form a resident council and have been unsuccessful, and if so, why. Also surveyors will look at other ways that residents and families can express grievances to administration.

A resident's or family group is defined as a group that meets regularly to:

- Discuss and offer suggestions about facility policies and procedures affecting residents' care, treatment, and quality of life;
- Support each other;

- Plan resident and family activities;
- Participate in educational activities; or
- For any other purpose.

CFR Section 483.15(c) Resident and Family Groups

(c) Participation in resident and family groups.

(1) A resident has the right to organize and participate in resident groups in the facility;
(2) A resident's family has the right to meet in the facility with the families of other residents in the facility;
(3) The facility must provide a resident or family group, if one exists, with private space;
(4) Staff or visitors may attend meetings at the group's invitation;
(5) The facility must provide a designated staff person responsible for providing assistance and responding to written requests that result from group meetings;
(6) When a resident or family group exists, the facility must listen to the views and act upon the grievances and recommendations of residents and families concerning proposed policy and operational decisions affecting resident care and life in the facility.

Interpretive Guidelines: Section 483.15(c) Resident/Family Council

This requirement does not require that residents organize a residents or family group. However, whenever residents or their families wish to organize, facilities must allow them to do so without interference. The facility must provide the group with space, privacy for meetings, and staff support. Normally, the designated staff person responsible for assistance and liaison between the group and the facility's administration and any other staff members attend the meeting only if requested.

The facility is required to listen to resident and family group recommendations and grievances. Acting upon these issues does not mean that the facility must accede to all group recommendations, but the facility must seriously consider the group's recommendations and must attempt to accommodate those recommendations, to the extent practicable, in developing and changing facility policies affecting resident care and life in the facility. The facility should communicate its decisions to the resident and/or family group.

B. Resident Group Interview

One of the significant tasks of the survey process is the resident group interview. If a resident and/or family council exists, the surveyors will meet with these groups for the interview task. Information from these interviews often prompts surveyors to investigate issues raised by the residents.

Documentation in a SNAP

The questions asked by the surveyors are actually a resident or family satisfaction survey. These same questions can be used by the facility for review with resident or family councils on a regular basis as part of the facility's Quality Assessment and Assurance program. By interviewing residents and families in this method, problems can be identified early and resolved quickly. Such interviews improve public relations and provide a feeling of control or empowerment for those involved in the interviews.

Resident Council President/Representative Interview

Council:

1. *Does the Resident Council meet on a regular basis?*
2. *Does the facility help with arrangements for council meetings?*
3. *Is there enough space for everyone who wants to attend?*
4. *Can you meet without staff present, if you desire?*

Grievances:

5. *Does staff listen to the resident's/Council's views and act upon any grievances the resident/group has filed?*
6. *Does appropriate facility staff respond to the resident's/group's concerns?*
7. *If the facility does not respond to concerns, do they give a reasonable explanation?*
8. *Do you feel a resident or the group can complain about care without worrying that someone will "get back" at them?*

Rules:

9. *Have you (residents) been informed of the rules at the facility (such as restrictions on visiting hours)?*
10. *Do you think the rules at this facility are fair to all residents?*

11. *If the Resident Council makes suggestions about some of the rules, does the facility act on those suggestions?*

Rights:

12. *Does staff talk about and review the rights of residents in the facility?*
13. *Are residents able to exercise their rights?*
14. *Do you feel that the rights of residents at this facility are respected and encouraged?*
15. *Is mail delivered unopened and on Saturdays?*
16. *Without having to ask, are the results of the State inspection available to read?*
17. *Do residents know who the ombudsman is and how to contact her/him?*
18. *Does the facility allow you to see your medical records if you ask?*
19. *Have residents been informed of their right (and given information on how) to formally complain to the State about the care they are receiving?*
20. *Do you have any questions, or is there anything else you would like to tell me about the Resident Council?*

It is recommended that these questions are periodically asked of the resident council to evaluate and identify problems. This could be done by taking on a set of questions for discussion at each monthly meeting.

C. Minutes

Meetings are most productive when effectively organized. The activity professional can assist the resident or family council in setting up an agenda prior to the meeting.

Minutes of resident and family councils are necessary for meetings to be meaningful. Writing the minutes may be part of the assistance provided by staff. The facility may offer this duty is part of the activity professional's job description.

Minutes should include:

- Date
- Time of meeting
- Names of persons attending
- Unresolved issues and status
- New concerns
- Follow-up to ongoing issues
- Signature of council president
- Signature of person taking the minute

SAMPLE NURSING FACILITY

MINUTES OF RESIDENT COUNCIL

Date: _____

The meeting was called to order by the Chairperson, (NAME), at (TIME) AM/PM.

The following residents attended this meeting:

The following staff members or guests were invited to attend the meeting:

The minutes of the previous meeting were reviewed and approved.

The following unresolved issues were discussed and reports were given of action taken in response to the issues raised by the Resident Council.

The following issues were resolved by (specify the action taken to resolve each issue).

The following issues were discussed and recommendations were made.

The meeting was adjourned at (TIME) AM/PM.

Respectfully submitted,

Secretary

SAMPLE NURSING FACILITY

MINUTES OF RESIDENT COUNCIL

FOR THE MONTH OF _____

PROBLEMS	ACTION	RESOLUTION

Submitted by _____, Activity Director

Reported to _____, Administrator

D. Action Summary

In addition to narrative minutes, a summary sheet to follow-up issues raised at the resident council is helpful to document that the facility has seriously considered any recommendations. This action summary should track the issues, actions taken, and follow-up.

EXAMPLE OF RESIDENT COUNCIL ACTION SUMMARY

Problems	Action	Resolution
Suggest birthday parties be held on weekends or evenings so families could attend.	Activity Director will survey families to determine most convenient time.	Report to January meeting on findings.
Request warm drinks for nourishments on winter afternoons in November through March.	Activity Director will contact the Dietary Supervisor to discuss. Possibility to purchase microwave discussed with Administrator.	Warm drinks are now available on Unit I. Microwave purchased in November. Unit II will have microwave in February.

10. QUALITY ASSESSMENT AND ASSURANCE

KEY POINTS AND SUMMARY OF CHAPTER

Quality Assessment and Assurance (QAA) is an ongoing program and not just a once a year crash effort to prepare for survey.

A Quality Assessment and Assurance program matches expected outcomes of care to actual practice to find opportunities for improvement.

Quality indicators (QI) are measurements of outcomes of care.

Audit checklists and satisfaction questionnaires are some of the tools used to identify problem areas the need to be improved.

The QAA program will be replaced sometime after 2012 with a Quality Assessment and Performance Improvement (QAPI) program. Some specifics may change, but the overall goals of improving quality are the same in both programs.

Quality Assessment and Assurance (QAA) is a continuous program that monitors the ability of a nursing facility to achieve positive outcomes of care. A QAA program matches expected outcomes of care to actual practice. When expectations are not met, staff is alerted that potential problems exist. An analysis of causal factors is done, and actions taken to improve performance.

The result of an effective quality assessment and assurance program is identification and resolution of problems before they become too large or too difficult to fix. Early identification of trends provides opportunities to improve resident care.

A. Federal Regulations

CMS has made a commitment not only to survey for compliance with regulations but also to improve the quality of care in nursing homes. MDS data is used to calculate quality indicators (QI) and quality measures (QM) that are used in the survey process. These indicators measure and identify potential areas of concern. Quality measures (QM) are also posted on the CMS website Nursing Home Compare. Consumers can access the site for information about nursing homes. The federal regulations require that nursing homes have a process to review and improve quality of care. Specifically, a Quality Assessment and Assurance (QAA) Committee must be functioning in the facility.

Some time after 2012 the QAA program will change to a Quality Assessment and Performance Improvement (QAPI) program. The exact structure and requirements of the new program were not known at the time this book was written.

CFR Section 483.75(o) Quality Assessment and Assurance Committee

(1) A facility must maintain a quality assessment and assurance committee consisting of
    (i) The director of nursing service;
    (ii) A physician designated by the facility;
    (iii) At least 3 other members of the facility staff.
(2) The quality assessment and assurance committee
    (i) Meets at least quarterly to identify issues with respect to which quality assessment and assurance activities are necessary; and
    (ii) Develops and implements appropriate plans of action to correct identified quality deficiencies.
(3) A State or the Secretary may not require disclosure of the records of such committee except in so far as such disclosure is related to the compliance of such committee with the requirements of this section.

During the survey process, the quality assessment and assurance protocol will be reviewed by the surveyor to determine that:

- A Quality Assessment and Assurance Committee exists and meets at least quarterly.
- The committee has a method, on a routine basis, to identify, respond to, and evaluate its response to issues that require quality assessment and assurance activity.

Because QAA reports and minutes are confidential, surveyors may not review the documentation. To determine that there is an effective QAA program, surveyors may ask QAA committee members and/or direct care staff questions about the QAA committee.

Direct care staff should know how to access the QAA process and committee. Access may be by participation on the committee or by submitting reports. Staff will attend inservice training in response to problems identified by QAA.

B. Implementation

To implement a Quality Assessment and Assurance (QAA) program, each facility must develop a system to measure actual performance and identify areas for improvement. A root analysis examines and identifies causes of the problem. Action is taken to correct any deficiencies found. And finally, the committee evaluates and follows up to assure that problems have been solved and quality improved.

Dr. W. Edward Deming was a pioneer in the development of quality assurance methods and performance improvement projects. His system outlined the following steps:

Plan: Study existing processes to decide if change will lead to improvement. Set a specific objective and measurable outcome to be attained. Identify who, what, where, when, and how the study will be done.

Do: Measure actual practice against expected practice outcomes. Identify problems and procedures that need change.

Study: Check and evaluate the results and draw conclusions.

Act: Implement policy and procedure changes. Monitor the changes. Train staff. Monitor the changes to assure improvement.

The Centers for Medicare and Medicaid Services (CMS) will develop best practices for a specific method for quality assessment and assurance. Best practices are proven methods to assure quality care. Any system used must identify when problems exist, identify causes and provide a way to correct the problems identified, thereby improving quality of care.

Review resident outcomes with the goal of improving care. Selection of issues to be studied in a performance improvement project should be made from objective data that measures outcomes of care. Gather information systematically to clarify issues or problems. Analyze information to determine the root cause of the problem. Develop interventions for improvement. Check and evaluate the results of changes and draw conclusions. Revise facility policies and procedures and train staff to do it right the first time. Re-evaluate outcome measurements and use recognized benchmarks to assess progress.

Resident and family satisfaction questionnaires are another way to identify problem areas. Use the resident and family councils as opportunities to gather information about resident and family concerns. Or ask families and residents to fill out a questionnaire at the time of discharge or annually to gather information about care.

Overall responsibility for QAA is assigned to a person within the facility designated as the Quality Assessment and Assurance Coordinator. This person's role is to assist each department to identify which aspects of care need to be monitored. The QAA Coordinator may help with development of clinical indicators, data collection, root analysis, and implementation of actions for correction.

STEPS IN A QUALITY ASSESSMENT AND ASSURANCE PROGRAM

1. Assign responsibility for QAA monitoring and commitment of administration
2. Identify the departments and staff to be involved
3. Target aspects of care to be studied on an ongoing basis
4. Develop objective measurements of the quality of care

5. Collect data of actual practice
6. Evaluate the information collected to clarify problem and determine root cause
7. Take systematic actions to correct problems identified
8. Determine whether corrective action was successful
9. Communicate actions to the governing body (administration)

C. Quality Indicators

Quality indicators are measurements that test the outcomes of the activity program. By using measurement devices, such as quality indicators, actual current practice in the facility can be described. The current practices are then evaluated and matched against expectations to identify areas that need improvement.

1. Types of Quality Indicators

There are various ways to look at outcomes of the activity program: Services, Resident Satisfaction, Regulations, Utilization of Services, Management, and Cost Analysis (Financial). Actual performance is measured against the quality indicator selected. The clinical indicators will identify the quality of the activity program.

TYPES AND EXAMPLES OF QUALITY INDICATORS

Type	Definition	Example
Services	Evaluation of services provided	*Number of residents with little or no activity participation*
Resident Satisfaction	Resident's perception of service	*Resident and Family Questionnaires will be "good" or "excellent"*
Regulatory	Legal requirements	*100% of residents will have a copy of the current activity calendar in their room*
Utilization	Volume of services	*75% of residents will attend an activity program 3 times a week*
Management	Productivity standards	*A minimum of three one-hour activity programs will be scheduled on weekends*
Financial	Cost analysis	*Increase intergenerational programs to one each month by adding at least two more kindergarten through eighth grade volunteer groups*

Services   Do the programs offered meet the needs of the current residents in the facility?

Resident Satisfaction	Are the residents happy with the programs or are there other programs that the resident's want that are not now available?
Regulations	Are federal regulations for activity services being met?
Utilization of Services	Does the activity program have enough programs at convenient times of the day and week to meet all residents' needs?
Management	Are residents transported to programs in a timely manner?
Cost Analysis	What is the cost of the programs to the facility?

2. Methods of Measuring Quality

Quality indicators can be measured by various tools. Measurement is done by observing, interviewing, auditing, or collecting data about the actual level of performance. All or any combination of these methods may be part of an effective QAA program.

Some methods of measuring quality are

- Statistical process control,
- Resident/Family Satisfaction Questionnaires,
- Suggestion Boxes, and
- Self-evaluation checklists.

When the actual performance or outcome of the activity program is below expectations, it is time to determine a root cause and areas for improvement. Plans to change or improve performance and outcomes are developed. Actions to correct the identified problem are begun.

Improvement plans can include:

- staff training,
- both inservice and continuing education,
- purchase or repair of equipment,
- reorganization of work flow, and/or
- revisions to policies and procedures.

Once an action plan has been completed, the results of the actions are then re-evaluated to determine actual performance according to the quality indicator. Do a follow up study to check that actions have resulted in quality improvement.

3. Examples of Quality Indicators and Thresholds

The federal government included in the survey process quality indicators based on MDS data that have been transmitted to CMS. These measurements allow surveyors to focus on target areas. Each quality indicator contains a measurement of a process or outcome of care and a threshold for action. The threshold for action is expressed by a number of times a specific outcome should occur or by a percentage of times that an outcome should be achieved.

EXAMPLES OF CLINICAL INDICATORS
WITH THRESHOLDS FOR ACTION

- Attendance at *(specific)* activity program should not be less than *(number)* of residents.
- Monthly there will be *(number)* of excursions outside the nursing facility for ambulatory residents.
- Monthly there will be *(number)* of excursions outside the nursing facility for non-ambulatory residents.
- Community groups will visit residents *(specify numbers)* times a week.
- Residents who do not or cannot attend group activities will have in-room visits daily.
- Positive response *(good or excellent)* on Resident Satisfaction questionnaire will be above 90%.
- Activity occur as scheduled on the activity calendar 90% of the time unless a notice of change has been posted 24 hours prior the change.
- Responses to recommendations of Resident or Family Council are completed and returned back to the council within three weeks of each meeting.

> DEFINITIONS
>
> **QUALITY INDICATOR**
> Objective and measurable statements of outcomes of care, staff performance, or resident response.
>
> **THRESHOLD FOR ACTION**
> The level or point at which care should be evaluated to determine if there is an actual problem or opportunity to improve resident care.

To achieve quality improvement, the QAA committee must carefully study and identify the root cause(s) for the quality indicator not being met.

Identification of possible causes needs to include:

- evaluation of the results of the monitoring and
- drawing appropriate conclusions that will lead to improvement.

Before changing policies or procedures or implementing corrective action, be sure that the correct causal factors have been identified. This may be done by trial or pilot projects on a limited scale to determine the effectiveness of the actions taken.

D. Data Collection

Once quality indicators have been agreed upon, the actual delivery of care is monitored. Additional paperwork is not always necessary. Data can be collected from flow sheets already available, such as activity attendance records, one-to-one visit records, or computer generated reports based on MDS data.

Checklists may be used for specific monitoring topics:

- resident/family satisfaction surveys,
- review of environmental needs of activity program,
- audit of the activity calendar,
- chart audit for required documentation, and
- minutes of resident or family council meetings.

Case review for residents with special needs such as hearing and vision impairment or language problems can be used to evaluate the prevalence of such cases or for tracking types of interventions that are most successful.

Other useful QAA monitoring tools are resident satisfaction surveys. A positive outcome of care is that the resident is satisfied with the services provided. Resident questionnaires can be completed individually, by interview, or in a group setting.

Discussion from family and resident council meetings is an excellent source of issues and problems for quality assurance monitoring. Resident and family satisfaction or frequency of complaints is a measurement of quality.

The customer is always right. This motto has special meaning particularly during the survey process. Surveyors are instructed to interview residents and family about the care provided at the facility. Complaints voiced during such interviews will be thoroughly investigated. An ongoing program of interviewing residents and families is an effective means of identifying problems, many that can be quickly and effortlessly resolved.

Suggestion boxes are sometimes used to collect input from staff or family who are not actively participating in any formal means of communicating their ideas. Also designating a Quality Assurance and Improvement Month with activities and celebrations of QAA accomplishments can increase awareness of the program among staff and stimulate success.

Forms that can be used to monitor resident satisfaction and the quality of the activity program environment are shown on the next two pages.

RESIDENT SATISFACTION QUESTIONNAIRE

Date: _____

Purpose: To evaluate the resident's satisfaction with the activity program.

Question	Response
1. Does the activity program meet your interests?	
2. Are there activities that interest you that are not available?	
3. Are you satisfied with the times activities are offered?	
4. Are you satisfied with the number of activities offered?	
5. Are you satisfied with the use of community resources?	
6. Is adequate assistance provided so that you can participate in programs?	
7. Does the activity program address your special needs?	

OTHER REMARKS:

RESIDENT NAME: _____

INTERVIEWED BY: _____

ACTIVITY PROGRAM ENVIRONMENTAL AUDIT

Date of Audit: _____ Auditor: _____

INDICATORS	YES	NO	N/A
1. Activity Calendar:			
a. Current activities calendar is posted in areas accessible to all residents and staff on each unit.			
b. Activity calendar is easy to read and offers a variety of programs.			
c. All activity calendars are retained for one year.			
2. Program Design:			
a. Activity programs are provided seven days a week.			
b. Evening activity programs are provided often enough to meet stated needs of residents.			
c. Residents unable to attend programs held in the activity area receive 1:1 contact at least once daily.			
3. Activities Area:			
a. Sufficient space provided in activities area to accommodate scheduled activities without restricting movement and/or active participation of residents.			
b. Furnishings are in good repair, clean, and at the proper height for activities.			
c. Areas are clean and maintained.			
d. Area is free of any electrical or other safety hazard.			
e. There is adequate lighting and ventilation.			
f. Lavatory is accessible to residents.			
g. Temperature is maintained at comfort level.			
4. Other			
a. Transportation of residents to/from programs is provided in a safe, organized, and timely manner.			
b. Resident's schedules (meals, meds, rehab therapy) are coordinated with the activity calendar.			

Comment on all "NO" answers:

Corrective action taken / follow up needed:

E. Activity Calendar Audit

Evaluation of the activity calendar to assure that it matches with the current resident case-mix is a logical starting point for QAA of Activity Programs. The residents currently in the facility should be reviewed to determine their unique needs. Start by categorizing residents according to their needs and preferences:

- Cognition, intact or deficit,
- Vision problems,
- Communication barriers,
- Hearing difficulties, and/or
- Language other than English

Customary routines such as:

- Goes outside at least 1x weekly,
- Tobacco use,
- Distinct food preferences,
- Cultural identification,
- Religious participation,
- Daily contact with friends/relatives, and/or
- Animal companions

Compile a profile of current residents based on their unique needs. Then review the current activity calendar to determine how many hours are offered weekly of activities suitable to resident's needs or customary routines and cultural/religious preferences. Forms to do this are shown on the next two pages.

Copies of activity calendars can be provided to each resident. Those programs that are suitable for the resident can be highlighted. This will assure that the resident and family are aware of those activities that the resident prefers or that will benefit the resident. The individualized calendar can also be used to make staff aware of those activities that the resident wishes to attend. Staff can remind the resident to attend or assist the resident by transporting him or her to those activities that are appropriate.

F. Audit Checklists

Checklists are tools for a self-evaluation process. Checklist audits should be done on a regular schedule to identify problems as early as possible. A form for conducting an audit is shown on the third page following. Auditing will not correct a problem but auditing will describe what the problem is. Auditing, however, must have follow-up. Identify those persons responsible for correcting an identified deficiency. Verify that deficiencies are corrected.

ACTIVITY PROGRAM — RESIDENT NEEDS

Date of Audit _____ Auditor _____

INSTRUCTIONS: List all the residents by name and room number. In each column indicate with a check mark any of the resident's special needs or preferences.

Resident Name Room Number	Cognition		Impaired		Non-English Language		Religion/Cultural Preferences		
	Intact	Deficit	Sight	Hearing	Spanish	Other	Catholic	Jewish	Other
Totals									

ACTIVITY PROGRAM — PROGRAM OFFERINGS

Date of Audit _____ Auditor _____

INSTRUCTIONS: List all activities in the first column. For each scheduled activity identify the number of hours each week that the activity is scheduled and list under as many headings as apply to that activity program.

Title of Activity Program	Cognition		Impaired		Non-English Language		Religion/Cultural Preferences		
	Intact	Deficit	Sight	Hearing	Spanish	Other	Catholic	Jewish	Other
Total hours per week									

ACTIVITY PROGRAM — CHART AUDIT

No. _____ Resident Name _____ Room _____

INDICATORS	YES	NO	N/A
1. **Assessment:** a. Completed within 7 days of admission			
b. Content includes current and past interests			
physical needs and abilities			
mental needs and abilities			
2. **Interdisciplinary Care Plan:** Completed on admission for welcome/orientation			
Comprehensive care plan addresses activity needs			
Identifies measurable objective goals			
Plan updated a. quarterly			
b. modified as needed			
3. **Progress Notes** Written at least quarterly			
Assess progress or regress to goals identified in care plan			

COMMENTS:

Date: _____ Audited by: _____

G. Corrective Action

Quality indicators that are not met alert staff that care should be evaluated to determine if there is an actual problem or opportunity to improve resident care. Unmet indicators do not always mean that quality of care is below standard. Further review of the actual activity program is required to determine the cause of declining attendance.

For example, a quality indicator could be that at least ten residents are present at the current events program every morning.

- The quality indicator is the attendance of residents at the current events program.
- The threshold for action is that at least ten residents should attend.

If the month's attendance is 15 or more residents, the clinical indicator is met. If, however, after several months, or during the month of December only, the attendance drops to below ten residents each morning, the quality indicator alerts the staff that something has changed.

Of course, the finding that attendance of an activity program has declined does not necessarily mean that it is a poor quality program. The reason for the change in attendance needs to be investigated and the cause identified. Only when the causal factors are identified can effective corrective action be accomplished. The threshold is an alert that something has changed.

For example, some causes after investigation might be

Two new nursing assistants were recently hired and are slow to bathe and dress residents in the morning delaying their leaving their rooms in time for the current events program.

Review of the types of residents that are in the nursing facility show a change to a larger number of bedfast residents, so that there are no longer ten residents available for whom this program would be suitable.

During the month of December a special Holiday Arts and Crafts volunteer conducts a class at the same time as the current events.

After determining the cause for the quality indicator not being met, actions are taken to correct the problem.

For example some actions could be

Nursing assistants' workload is evaluated by the Director of Nurses and adjustment made so that residents who wish to attend the current events program receive morning care first or early enough to attend the program.

Since there are no longer ten residents who are able to attend the current events program, the clinical indicator can be adjusted to a lower number to reflect the actual needs of the resident population. Additionally, the activity program calendar is re-evaluated to develop programs that would meet the needs of the current residents, such as more in-room programs for bedfast residents.

No changes are indicated in the program, since the Holiday Arts and Crafts was a once a year program by a volunteer. If necessary, a change in time of the current events program for the month of December would allow the residents who attend the arts and crafts to also attend the current events.

H. Follow-up of Actions Taken

Summary reports of the QAA process must include problems identified, assessment of causes, corrective actions planned, results of interventions, and a re-evaluation of current performance. The form on the next page is one way to track corrective actions taken.

Narrative summary reports should be completed by department staff or the QAA Coordinator to track issues identified by the quality assessment and assurance process. The time and effort in assessing practice must be followed with actions taken to improve performance. The documentation should track the problems identified, actions taken, and follow up.

EXAMPLES OF ACTION FOLLOW UP

PROBLEMS	ACTION	RESOLUTION
Decline in attendance at 10:00 AM current events program during the month of December only	Conflicts with Holiday Arts and Crafts, change to 4:00	December attendance back to 10 to 15 residents now that time has changed for this month only
Activity program calendar changed 5 times this month	Last minute changes for Christmas Singers to avoid conflicts	Before Thanksgiving, confirm as many as possible (75%) of special Christmas visits with outside volunteers

QUALITY ASSESSMENT AND ASSURANCE

SUMMARY REPORT OF CORRECTIVE ACTIONS

For the meeting of _____

PROBLEMS	ACTION	RESOLUTION

Date _____ Submitted by _____

I. Departmental Preparation

Quality assessment and assurance applies to every department in the nursing facility. Desired outcomes of care are identified. Clinical indicators that measure actual practice are developed and/or approved by each department. If QAA is to work, staff participation is essential. Staff must agree to the standards against which their services will be measured.

All departments report quarterly to the Quality Assessment and Assurance Committee about their monitoring activities. These reports are made a part of the QAA minutes with copies to the administrator.

Quarterly reports summarize the monitoring activities:

- the problems identified,
- the investigation of the causes, and
- the corrective action taken

The forms on the next two pages show examples of how to report monitoring that has been done on activity programs.

QUALITY ASSESSMENT AND ASSURANCE REPORT FORM

DEPARTMENT: Activity Program   For the months of _____

QUALITY INDICATORS

1.   Ambulatory residents will have weekly excursions outside facility.

2.   Non-ambulatory residents will have monthly excursions outside facility.

3.   Volunteer groups from the community will be scheduled for visits twice a week.

4.   At least fifteen residents will attend Resident Council.

MONTHS OF			
Number of excursions outside facility for: Ambulatory residents			
Non-ambulatory residents			
Attendance at Resident Council (Number of Attendees)			
Number of visits from community groups Religious			
Intergenerational			
Special therapy			
Other:			
Number of residents with 1:1 visits By volunteers			
By activity program staff			

COMMENTS:

Dated _____ Submitted By _____

QUALITY ASSESSMENT AND ASSURANCE REPORT FORM

DEPARTMENT: Activity Program   For the months of _____

Problems identified by Audit Tools _____

_____

_____

_____

Problems identified from Resident Satisfaction Surveys _____

_____

_____

_____

Problems identified in Resident or Family Council _____

_____

_____

_____

New Policies and Procedures _____

_____

_____

_____

_____

_____

Dated _____ Submitted by _____

APPENDICES

Appendix A.
Federal Regulations (for activities) (State Operations Manual 100)

State Operations Manual 100-7 Appendix PP

F248 §483.15(f) Activities

§483.15(f)(1) The facility must provide for an ongoing program of activities designed to meet, in accordance with the comprehensive assessment, the interests and the physical, mental, and psychosocial wellbeing of each resident.

INTENT: §483.15(f)(1) Activities

The intent of this requirement is that:

- The facility identifies each resident's interests and needs; and
- The facility involves the resident in an ongoing program of activities that is designed to appeal to his or her interests and to enhance the resident's highest practicable level of physical, mental, and psychosocial well-being.

DEFINITIONS

Definitions are provided to clarify key terms used in this guidance.

- "Activities" refer to any endeavor, other than routine ADLs, in which a resident participates that is intended to enhance her/his sense of well-being and to promote or enhance physical, cognitive, and emotional health. These include, but are not limited to, activities that promote self-esteem, pleasure, comfort, education, creativity, success, and independence.

  NOTE: ADL-related activities, such as manicures/pedicures, hair styling, and makeovers, may be considered part of the activities program.

- "One-to-One Programming" refers to programming provided to residents who will not, or cannot, effectively plan their own activity pursuits, or residents needing specialized or extended programs to enhance their overall daily routine and activity pursuit needs.
- "Person Appropriate" refers to the idea that each resident has a personal identity and history that involves more than just their medical illnesses or functional impairments. Activities should be relevant to the specific needs, interests, culture, background, etc. of the individual for whom they are developed.
- "Program of Activities" includes a combination of large and small group, one-to-one, and self-directed activities; and a system that supports the development, implementation, and evaluation of the activities provided to the residents in the facility. [1]

OVERVIEW

In long term care, an ongoing program of activities refers to the provision of activities in accordance with and based upon an individual resident's comprehensive assessment. The Institute of Medicine (IOM)'s 1986 report, "Improving the Quality of Care in Nursing Homes," became the basis for the "Nursing Home Reform" part of OBRA '87 and the current OBRA long term care regulations. The IOM Report identified the need for residents in nursing homes to receive care and/or services to maximize their highest practicable quality of life. However, defining "quality of life" has been difficult, as it is subjective for each person. Thus, it is important for the facility to conduct an individualized assessment of each resident to provide additional opportunities to help enhance a resident's self-esteem and dignity.

Research findings and the observations of positive resident outcomes confirm that activities are an integral component of residents' lives. Residents have indicated that daily life and involvement should be meaningful. Activities are meaningful when they reflect a person's interests and lifestyle, are enjoyable to the person, help the person to feel useful, and provide a sense of belonging. [2]

Residents' Views on Activities

Activities are relevant and valuable to residents' quality of life. In a large-scale study commissioned by CMS, 160 residents in 40 nursing homes were interviewed about what quality of life meant to them. The study found that residents "overwhelmingly assigned priority to dignity, although they labeled this concern in many ways." The researchers determined that the two main components of dignity, in the words of these residents, were "independence" and "positive self-image." Residents listed, under the categories of independence and positive self-image, the elements of "choice of activities" and "activities that amount to something," such as those that produce or teach something; activities using skills from residents' former work; religious activities; and activities that contribute to the nursing home.

The report stated that, "Residents not only discussed particular activities that gave them a sense of purpose but also indicated that a lack of appropriate activities contributes to having no sense of purpose." "Residents rarely mentioned participating in activities as a way to just 'keep busy' or just to socialize... The relevance of the activities to the residents' lives must be considered."

According to the study, residents wanted a variety of activities, including those that are not childish, require thinking (such as word games), are gender-specific, produce something useful, relate to previous work of residents, allow for socializing with visitors and participating in community events, and are physically active. The study found that the above concepts were relevant to both interviewable and non-interviewable residents. Researchers observed that non-interviewable residents appeared "happier" and "less agitated" in homes with many planned activities for them.

Non-traditional Approaches to Activities

Surveyors need to be aware that some facilities may take a non-traditional approach to activities. In neighborhoods/households, all staff may be trained as nurse aides and are responsible to provide activities, and activities may resemble those of a private home. [3] Residents, staff, and families may interact in ways that reflect daily life, instead of in formal activities programs. Residents may be more involved in the ongoing activities in their living area, such as care-planned approaches including chores, preparing foods, meeting with other residents to choose spontaneous activities, and leading an activity. It has been reported that, "some culture changed homes might not have a traditional activities calendar, and instead focus on community life to include activities." Instead of an "activities director," some homes have a Community Life Coordinator, a Community Developer, or other title for the individual directing the activities program. [4]

For more information on activities in homes changing to a resident-directed culture, the following websites are available as resources: www.pioneernetwork.net; www.culturechangenow.com; www.qualitypartnersri.org (click on nursing homes); and www.edenalt.com.

ASSESSMENT

The information gathered through the assessment process should be used to develop the activities component of the comprehensive care plan. The ongoing program of activities should match the skills, abilities, needs, and preferences of each resident with the demands of the activity and the characteristics of the physical, social, and cultural environments. [5]

In order to develop individualized care planning goals and approaches, the facility should obtain sufficient, detailed information (even if the Activities RAP is not triggered) to determine what activities the resident prefers and what adaptations, if any, are needed. [6] The facility may use, but need not duplicate, information from other sources, such as the RAI, including the RAPs, assessments by other disciplines, observation, and resident and family interviews. Other sources of relevant information include the resident's lifelong interests, spirituality, life roles, goals, strengths, needs, and activity pursuit patterns and preferences. [7] This assessment should be completed by or under the supervision of a qualified professional (see F249 for definition of qualified professional).

> NOTE: Some residents may be independently capable of pursuing their own activities without intervention from the facility. This information should be noted in the assessment and identified in the plan of care.

CARE PLANNING

Care planning involves identification of the resident's interests, preferences, and abilities; and any issues, concerns, problems, or needs affecting the resident's involvement/engagement in activities. [8] In addition to the activities component of the comprehensive care plan, information may also be found in a separate activity plan, on a CNA flow sheet, in a progress note, etc.

Activity goals related to the comprehensive care plan should be based on measurable objectives and focused on desired outcomes (e.g., engagement in an activity that matches the resident's ability, maintaining attention to the activity for a specified period of time, expressing satisfaction with the activity verbally or non-verbally), not merely on attendance at a certain number of activities per week.

> NOTE: For residents with no discernable response, service provision is still expected and may include one-to-one activities such as talking to the

resident, reading to the resident about prior interests, or applying lotion while stroking the resident's hands or feet.

Activities can occur at any time, are not limited to formal activities being provided only by activities staff, and can include activities provided by other facility staff, volunteers, visitors, residents, and family members. All relevant departments should collaborate to develop and implement an individualized activities program for each resident.

Some medications, such as diuretics, or conditions such as pain, incontinence, etc. may affect the resident's participation in activities. Therefore, additional steps may be needed to facilitate the resident's participation in activities, such as:

- If not contraindicated, timing the administration of medications, to the extent possible, to avoid interfering with the resident's ability to participate or to remain at a scheduled activity; or
- If not contraindicated, modifying the administration time of pain medication to allow the medication to take effect prior to an activity the resident enjoys.

The care plan should also identify the discipline(s) that will carry out the approaches. For example:

- Notifying residents of preferred activities;
- Transporting residents who need assistance to and from activities (including indoor, outdoor, and outings);
- Providing needed functional assistance (such as toileting and eating assistance); and
- Providing needed supplies or adaptations, such as obtaining and returning audio books, setting up adaptive equipment, etc.

Concepts the facility should have considered in the development of the activities component of the resident's comprehensive care plan include the following, as applicable to the resident:

- A continuation of life roles, consistent with resident preferences and functional capacity (e.g., to continue work or hobbies such as cooking, table setting, repairing small appliances) [9];
- Encouraging and supporting the development of new interests, hobbies, and skills (e.g., training on using the Internet); and
- Connecting with the community, such as places of worship, veterans' groups, volunteer groups, support groups, wellness groups, athletic or educational connections (via outings or invitations to outside groups to visit the facility).

The facility may need to consider accommodations in schedules, supplies, and timing in order to optimize a resident's ability to participate in an activity of choice. Examples of accommodations may include, but are not limited to:

- Altering a therapy or a bath/shower schedule to make it possible for a resident to attend a desired activity that occurs at the same time as the therapy session or bath;
- Assisting residents, as needed, to get to and participate in desired activities (e.g., dressing, toileting, transportation);

- Providing supplies (e.g., books/magazines, music, craft projects, cards, sorting materials) for activities, and assistance when needed, for residents' use (e.g., during weekends, nights, holidays, evenings, or when the activities staff are unavailable); and
- Providing a late breakfast to allow a resident to continue a lifelong pattern of attending religious services before eating.

INTERVENTIONS

The concept of individualized intervention has evolved over the years. Many activity professionals have abandoned generic interventions such as "reality orientation" and large-group activities that include residents with different levels of strengths and needs. In their place, individualized interventions have been developed based upon the assessment of the resident's history, preferences, strengths, and needs. These interventions have changed from the idea of "age-appropriate" activities to promoting "person-appropriate" activities. For example, one person may care for a doll or stroke a stuffed animal, another person may be inclined to reminisce about dolls or stuffed animals they once had, while someone else may enjoy petting a dog but will not be interested in inanimate objects. The surveyor observing these interventions should determine if the facility selected them in response to the resident's history and preferences. Many activities can be adapted in various ways to accommodate the resident's change in functioning due to physical or cognitive limitations.

Some Possible Adaptations that May be Made by the Facility [10, 11]

When evaluating the provision of activities, it is important for the surveyor to identify whether the resident has conditions and/or issues for which staff should have provided adaptations. Examples of adaptations for specific conditions include, but are not limited to the following:

- For the resident with visual impairments: higher levels of lighting without glare; magnifying glasses, light-filtering lenses, telescopic glasses; use of "clock method" to describe where items are located; description of sizes, shapes, colors; large print items including playing cards, newsprint, books; audio books;
- For the resident with hearing impairments: small group activities; placement of resident near speaker/activity leader; use of amplifiers or headphones; decreased background noise; written instructions; use of gestures or sign language to enhance verbal communication; adapted TV (closed captioning, magnified screen, earphones);
- For the resident who has physical limitations, the use of adaptive equipment, proper seating and positioning, placement of supplies and materials [12] (based on clinical assessment and referral as appropriate) to enhance:
  o Visual interaction and to compensate for loss of visual field (hemianopsia);
  o Upper extremity function and range of motion (reach);
  o Hand dexterity (e.g., adapted size of items such as larger handles for cooking and woodworking equipment, built-up paintbrush handles, large needles for crocheting);

o The ability to manipulate an item based upon the item's weight, such as lighter weight for residents with muscle weakness [13];

- For the resident who has the use of only one hand: holders for kitchen items, magazines/books, playing cards; items (e.g., art work, bingo card, nail file) taped to the table; c-clamp or suction vise to hold wood for sanding;
- For the resident with cognitive impairment: task segmentation and simplification; programs using retained long-term memory, rather than short-term memory; length of activities based on attention span; settings that recreate past experiences or increase/decrease stimulation; smaller groups without interruption; one-to-one activities;

NOTE: The length, duration, and content of specific one-to-one activities are determined by the specific needs of the individual resident, such as several short interventions (rather than a few longer activities) if someone has extremely low tolerance or if there are behavioral issues. Examples of one-to-one activities may include any of the following:

o Sensory stimulation or cognitive therapy (e.g., touch/visual/auditory stimulation, reminiscence, or validation therapy) such as special stimulus rooms or equipment; alerting/upbeat music and using alerting aromas or providing fabrics or other materials of varying textures;
o Social engagement (e.g., directed conversation, initiating a resident to resident conversation, pleasure walk, or coffee visit);
o Spiritual support, nurturing (e.g., daily devotion, Bible reading, or prayer with or for resident per religious requests/desires);
o Creative, task-oriented activities (e.g., music or pet activities/therapy, letter writing, word puzzles); or
o Support of self-directed activity (e.g., delivering of library books, craft material to rooms, setting up talking book service).

- For the resident with a language barrier: translation tools; translators; or publications and/or audio/video materials in the resident's language;
- For residents who are terminally ill: life review; quality time with chosen relatives, friends, staff, and/or other residents; spiritual support; touch; massage; music; and/or reading to the resident; [8]

NOTE: Some residents may prefer to spend their time alone and introspectively. Their refusal of activities does not necessarily constitute noncompliance.

- For the resident with pain: spiritual support, relaxation programs, music, massage, aromatherapy, pet therapy/pet visits, and/or touch;
- For the resident who prefers to stay in her/his own room or is unable to leave her/his room: in-room visits by staff/other residents/volunteers with similar interests/hobbies; touch and sensory activities such as massage or aromatherapy; access to art/craft materials, cards, games, reading materials; access to technology

of interest (computer, DVD, hand held video games, preferred radio programs/stations, audio books); and/or visits from spiritual counselors; [14]

- For the resident with varying sleep patterns, activities are available during awake time. Some facilities use a variety of options when activities staff are not available for a particular resident: nursing staff reads a newspaper with resident; dietary staff makes finger foods available; CNA works puzzle with the resident; maintenance staff take the resident on night rounds; and/or early morning delivery of coffee/juice to residents;
- For the resident who has recently moved in: welcoming activities and/or orientation activities;
- For the short-stay resident: "a la carte activities" are available, such as books, magazines, cards, word puzzles, newspapers, CDs, movies, and handheld games; interesting/contemporary group activities are offered, such as dominoes, bridge, Pinochle, poker, video games, movies, and travelogues; and/or individual activities designed to match the goals of therapy, such as jigsaw puzzles to enhance fine motor skills;
- For the younger resident: individual and group music offerings that fit the resident's taste and era; magazines, books, and movies that fit the resident's taste and era; computer and Internet access; and/or contemporary group activities, such as video games, and the opportunity to play musical instruments, card and board games, and sports; and
- For residents from diverse ethnic or cultural backgrounds: special events that include meals, decorations, celebrations, or music; visits from spiritual leaders and other individuals of the same ethnic background; printed materials (newspapers, magazines) about the resident's culture; and/or opportunities for the resident and family to share information about their culture with other residents, families, and staff.

Activity Approaches for Residents with Behavioral Symptoms [15, 7]

When the surveyor is evaluating the activities provided to a resident who has behavioral symptoms, they may observe that many behaviors take place at about the same time every day (e.g., before lunch or mid-afternoon). The facility may have identified a resident's pattern of behavior symptoms and may offer activity interventions, whenever possible, prior to the behavior occurring. Once a behavior escalates, activities may be less effective or may even cause further stress to the resident (some behaviors may be appropriate reactions to feelings of discomfort, pain, or embarrassment, such as aggressive behaviors exhibited by some residents with dementia during bathing [16]). Examples of activities-related interventions that a facility may provide to try to minimize distressed behavior may include, but are not limited to the following:

For the resident who is constantly walking:

- Providing a space and environmental cues that encourages physical exercise, decreases exit behavior, and reduces extraneous stimulation (such as seating areas spaced along a walking path or garden; a setting in which the resident may manipulate objects; or a room with a calming atmosphere, for example, using music, light, and rocking chairs);

- Providing aroma(s)/aromatherapy that is/are pleasing and calming to the resident; and
- Validating the resident's feelings and words; engaging the resident in conversation about who or what they are seeking; and using one-to-one activities, such as reading to the resident or looking at familiar pictures and photo albums.

For the resident who engages in name-calling, hitting, kicking, yelling, biting, sexual behavior, or compulsive behavior:

- Providing a calm, non-rushed environment, with structured, familiar activities such as folding, sorting, and matching; using one-to-one activities or small group activities that comfort the resident, such as their preferred music, walking quietly with the staff, a family member, or a friend; eating a favorite snack; looking at familiar pictures;
- Engaging in exercise and movement activities; and
- Exchanging self-stimulatory activity for a more socially appropriate activity that uses the hands, if in a public space.

For the resident who disrupts group activities with behaviors such as talking loudly and being demanding, or the resident who has catastrophic reactions such as uncontrolled crying or anger, or the resident who is sensitive to too much stimulation:

- Offering activities in which the resident can succeed, that are broken into simple steps, that involve small groups or are one-to-one activities such as using the computer, that are short and repetitive, and that are stopped if the resident becomes overwhelmed (reducing excessive noise such as from the television);
- Involving in familiar occupation-related activities. (A resident, if they desire, can do paid or volunteer work and the type of work would be included in the resident's plan of care, such as working outside the facility, sorting supplies, delivering resident mail, passing juice and snacks, refer to F169, Work);
- Involving in physical activities such as walking, exercise or dancing, games or projects requiring strategy, planning, and concentration, such as model building, and creative programs such as music, art, dance or physically resistive activities, such as kneading clay, hammering, scrubbing, sanding, using a punching bag, using stretch bands, or lifting weights; and
- Slow exercises (e.g., slow tapping, clapping, or drumming); rocking or swinging motions (including a rocking chair).

For the resident who goes through others' belongings:

- Using normalizing activities such as stacking canned food onto shelves, folding laundry; offering sorting activities (e.g., sorting socks, ties, or buttons); involving in organizing tasks (e.g., putting activity supplies away); providing rummage areas in plain sight, such as a dresser; and
- Using non-entry cues, such as "Do not disturb" signs or removable sashes, at the doors of other residents' rooms; providing locks to secure other resident's belongings (if requested).

For the resident who has withdrawn from previous activity interests/customary routines and isolates self in room/bed most of the day:

Documentation in a SNAP

- Providing activities just before or after meal time and where the meal is being served (out of the room);
- Providing in-room volunteer visits, music, or videos of choice;
- Encouraging volunteer-type work that begins in the room and needs to be completed outside of the room, or a small group activity in the resident's room, if the resident agrees; working on failure-free activities, such as simple structured crafts or other activity with a friend; having the resident assist another person;
- Inviting to special events with a trusted peer or family/friend;
- Engaging in activities that give the resident a sense of value (e.g., intergenerational activities that emphasize the resident's oral history knowledge);
- Inviting resident to participate on facility committees;
- Inviting the resident outdoors; and
- Involving in gross motor exercises (e.g., aerobics, light weight training) to increase energy and uplift mood.

For the resident who excessively seeks attention from staff and/or peers:

- Including in social programs, small group activities, service projects, with opportunities for leadership.

For the resident who lacks awareness of personal safety, such as putting foreign objects in her/his mouth or who is self-destructive and tries to harm self by cutting or hitting self, head banging, or causing other injuries to self:

- Observing closely during activities, taking precautions with materials (e.g., avoiding sharp objects and small items that can be put into the mouth);
- Involving in smaller groups or one-to-one activities that use the hands (e.g., folding towels, putting together PVC tubing);
- Focusing attention on activities that are emotionally soothing, such as listening to music or talking about personal strengths and skills, followed by participation in related activities; and
- Focusing attention on physical activities, such as exercise.

For the resident who has delusional and hallucinatory behavior that is stressful to her/him:

- Focusing the resident on activities that decrease stress and increase awareness of actual surroundings, such as familiar activities and physical activities; offering verbal reassurance, especially in terms of keeping the resident safe; and acknowledging that the resident's experience is real to her/him.

The outcome for the resident, the decrease or elimination of the behavior, either validates the activity intervention or suggests the need for a new approach.

ENDNOTES

[1] Miller, M. E., Peckham, C. W., & Peckham, A. B. (1998). *Activities keep me going and going* (pp. 217-224). Lebanon, OH: Otterbein Homes.

[2] Alzheimer's Association (n.d.). Activity based Alzheimer care: Building a therapeutic program. Training presentation made 1998.

[3] Thomas, W. H. (2003). Evolution of Eden. In A. S. Weiner & J. L. Ronch (Eds.), *Culture change in long-term care* (pp. 146-157). New York: Haworth Press.

[4] Bowman, C. S. (2005). Living Life to the Fullest: A match made in OBRA '87. Milwaukee, WI: Action Pact, Inc.

[5] Glantz, C. G. & Richman, N. (2001). Leisure activities. In *Occupational therapy: Practice skills for physical dysfunction*. St Louis: Mosby.

[6] Glantz, C. G. & Richman, N. (1996). *Evaluation and intervention for leisure activities, ROTE: Role of Occupational Therapy for the Elderly* (2nd ed., p. 728). Bethesda, MD.: American Occupational Therapy Association.

[7] Glantz, C. G. & Richman, N. (1998). *Creative methods, materials and models for training trainers in Alzheimer's education* (pp. 156-159). Riverwoods, IL: Glantz/Richman Rehabilitation Associates.

[8] Hellen, C. (1992). *Alzheimer's disease: Activity-focused care* (pp. 128-130). Boston, MA: Andover.

[9] American Occupational Therapy Association. (2002). Occupational therapy practice framework: domain & process. *American Journal of Occupational Therapy, 56*(6), 616-617. Bethesda, MD: American Occupational Therapy Association.

[10] Henderson, A., Cermak, S., Costner, W., Murray, E., Trombly, C., & Tickle-Gegnen, L. (1991). The issue is: Occupational science is multidimensional. *American Journal of Occupational Therapy, 45*, 370-372, Bethesda, MD: American Occupational Therapy Association.

[11] Pedretti, L. W. (1996). Occupational performance: A model for practice in physical dysfunction. In L. W. Pedretti (Ed.), *Occupational therapy: Practice skills for physical dysfunction* (4th ed., pp. 3-11). St. Louis: Mosby-Year Book

[12] Christenson, M. A. (1996). *Environmental design, modification, and adaptation, ROTE: Role of occupational therapy for the elderly* (2nd ed., pp. 380-408). Bethesda, MD: American Occupational Therapy Association.

[13] Coppard, B. M., Higgins, T., & Harvey, K. D. (2004). Working with elders who have orthopedic conditions. In S. Byers-Connon, H. L. Lohman, and R. L. Padilla (Eds.), *Occupational therapy with elders: Strategies for the COTA* (2nd ed., p. 293). St. Louis, MO: Elsevier Mosby.

[14] Glantz, C. G. & Richman, N. (1992). *Activity programming for the resident with mental illness* (pp. 53-76). Riverwoods, IL: Glantz/Richman Rehabilitation Associates.

[15] Day, K. & Calkins, M. P. (2002). Design and dementia. In R. B. Bechtel & A. Churchman (Eds.), *Handbook of environmental psychology* (pp. 374-393). New York: Wiley.

[16] Barrick, A. L., Rader, J., Hoeffer, B., & Sloane, P. (2002). *Bathing without a battle: Personal care of individuals with dementia* (p. 4). New York: Springer.

Appendix B.
Copy of MDS Comprehensive

Facilities in the United States that receive Medicare funds are required to use a specific, standardized assessment on every resident admitted to the facility. This standardized assessment, called the Minimum Data Set (MDS), is an interdisciplinary assessment. Each member of the interdisciplinary team is required to conduct his/her own assessment of the resident, analyze the resident's status, and then summarize that information on the MDS form within 14 days of the resident's admission to the facility.

The MDS provides health care workers in long-term care settings with two advantages: 1. it standardizes medical vocabulary across the nation and 2. it provides the mechanism for the collection of information: demographic information, mortality and morbidity statistics, and treatment outcomes. The MDS has been used long enough for us to be able to recognize when a "score" on the MDS indicates health or when it indicates the need to provide some kind of treatment. A book that is used with the MDS, called *Resident Assessment System for Long-term Care*, outlines which scores or combination of scores point up the need for specific interventions.

The comprehensive MDS 3.0 report form is shown in this appendix.

MINIMUM DATA SET (MDS) - Version 3.0
RESIDENT ASSESSMENT AND CARE SCREENING
Nursing Home Comprehensive (NC) Item Set

Section A	Identification Information

A0050. Type of Record

Enter Code ☐

1. **Add new record** → Continue to A0100, Facility Provider Numbers
2. **Modify existing record** → Continue to A0100, Facility Provider Numbers
3. **Inactivate existing record** → Skip to X0150, Type of Provider

A0100. Facility Provider Numbers

A. National Provider Identifier (NPI):

☐☐☐☐☐☐☐☐☐☐

B. CMS Certification Number (CCN):

☐☐☐☐☐☐☐☐☐☐☐☐

C. State Provider Number:

☐☐☐☐☐☐☐☐☐☐☐☐☐☐

A0200. Type of Provider

Enter Code ☐

Type of provider
1. **Nursing home (SNF/NF)**
2. **Swing Bed**

A0310. Type of Assessment

Enter Code ☐☐

A. Federal OBRA Reason for Assessment
01. **Admission** assessment (required by day 14)
02. **Quarterly** review assessment
03. **Annual** assessment
04. **Significant change in status** assessment
05. **Significant correction** to **prior comprehensive** assessment
06. **Significant correction** to **prior quarterly** assessment
99. **None of the above**

Enter Code ☐☐

B. PPS Assessment
PPS Scheduled Assessments for a Medicare Part A Stay
01. **5-day** scheduled assessment
02. **14-day** scheduled assessment
03. **30-day** scheduled assessment
04. **60-day** scheduled assessment
05. **90-day** scheduled assessment
06. **Readmission/return** assessment
PPS Unscheduled Assessments for a Medicare Part A Stay
07. **Unscheduled assessment used for PPS** (OMRA, significant or clinical change, or significant correction assessment)
Not PPS Assessment
99. **None of the above**

Enter Code ☐

C. PPS Other Medicare Required Assessment - OMRA
0. **No**
1. **Start of therapy** assessment
2. **End of therapy** assessment
3. **Both Start and End of therapy** assessment
4. **Change of therapy** assessment

Enter Code ☐

D. Is this a Swing Bed clinical change assessment? Complete only if A0200 = 2
0. **No**
1. **Yes**

A0310 continued on next page

Section A	Identification Information

A0310. Type of Assessment - Continued

Enter Code	E. Is this assessment the first assessment (OBRA, Scheduled PPS, or Discharge) **since the most recent admission/entry or reentry?**
[ ]	0. **No** 1. **Yes**

Enter Code	F. Entry/discharge reporting
[ ][ ]	01. **Entry** tracking record 10. **Discharge** assessment-**return not anticipated** 11. **Discharge** assessment-**return anticipated** 12. **Death in facility** tracking record 99. **None of the above**

Enter Code	G. Type of discharge - Complete only if A0310F = 10 or 11
[ ]	1. **Planned** 2. **Unplanned**

A0410. Submission Requirement

Enter Code	1. **Neither federal nor state required submission** 2. **State but not federal required submission** (FOR NURSING HOMES ONLY) 3. **Federal required submission**
[ ]	

A0500. Legal Name of Resident

A. First name:

[ ][ ][ ][ ][ ][ ][ ][ ][ ][ ][ ][ ][ ][ ]

B. Middle initial:

[ ]

C. Last name:

[ ][ ][ ][ ][ ][ ][ ][ ][ ][ ][ ][ ][ ][ ][ ][ ][ ]

D. Suffix:

[ ][ ][ ]

A0600. Social Security and Medicare Numbers

A. Social Security Number:

[ ][ ][ ] – [ ][ ] – [ ][ ][ ][ ]

B. Medicare number (or comparable railroad insurance number):

[ ][ ][ ][ ][ ][ ][ ][ ][ ][ ][ ][ ]

A0700. Medicaid Number - Enter "+" if pending, "N" if not a Medicaid recipient

[ ][ ][ ][ ][ ][ ][ ][ ][ ][ ][ ][ ][ ][ ][ ]

A0800. Gender

Enter Code	1. **Male** 2. **Female**
[ ]	

A0900. Birth Date

[ ][ ] – [ ][ ] – [ ][ ][ ][ ]

Month   Day   Year

A1000. Race/Ethnicity

↓ Check all that apply

[ ]	A. **American Indian or Alaska Native**
[ ]	B. **Asian**
[ ]	C. **Black or African American**
[ ]	D. **Hispanic or Latino**
[ ]	E. **Native Hawaiian or Other Pacific Islander**
[ ]	F. **White**

MDS 3.0 Nursing Home Comprehensive (NC) Version 1.10.3 Effective 04/01/2012

Section A	Identification Information

A1100. Language

Enter Code	**A. Does the resident need or want an interpreter to communicate with a doctor or health care staff?**
☐	0. **No**
	1. **Yes** → Specify in A1100B, Preferred language
	9. **Unable to determine**

B. Preferred language:

☐☐☐☐☐☐☐☐☐☐☐☐☐☐☐☐

A1200. Marital Status

Enter Code	1. **Never married**
☐	2. **Married**
	3. **Widowed**
	4. **Separated**
	5. **Divorced**

A1300. Optional Resident Items

A. Medical record number:

☐☐☐☐☐☐☐☐☐☐☐☐

B. Room number:

☐☐☐☐☐☐☐☐☐

C. Name by which resident prefers to be addressed:

☐☐☐☐☐☐☐☐☐☐☐☐☐☐☐☐☐☐☐☐☐☐☐

D. Lifetime occupation(s) - put "/" between two occupations:

☐☐☐☐☐☐☐☐☐☐☐☐☐☐☐☐☐☐☐☐☐☐☐☐☐

A1500. Preadmission Screening and Resident Review (PASRR)
Complete only if A0310A = 01, 03, 04, or 05

Enter Code	**Is the resident currently considered by the state level II PASRR process to have serious mental illness and/or mental retardation or a related condition?**
☐	0. **No** → Skip to A1550, Conditions Related to MR/DD Status
	1. **Yes** → Continue to A1510, Level II Preadmission Screening and Resident Review (PASRR) Conditions
	9. **Not a Medicaid-certified unit** → Skip to A1550, Conditions Related to MR/DD Status

A1510. Level II Preadmission Screening and Resident Review (PASRR) Conditions
Complete only if A0310A = 01, 03, 04, or 05

	↓ Check all that apply
☐	A. Serious mental illness
☐	B. Mental Retardation
☐	C. Other related conditions

Section A	Identification Information

A1550. Conditions Related to MR/DD Status

If the resident is 22 years of age or older, complete only if A0310A = 01

If the resident is 21 years of age or younger, complete only if A0310A = 01, 03, 04, or 05

↓ Check all conditions that are related to MR/DD status that were manifested before age 22, and are likely to continue indefinitely

	MR/DD With Organic Condition
☐	A. Down syndrome
☐	B. Autism
☐	C. Epilepsy
☐	D. Other organic condition related to MR/DD
	MR/DD Without Organic Condition
☐	E. MR/DD with no organic condition
	No MR/DD
☐	Z. None of the above

A1600. Entry Date (date of this admission/entry or reentry into the facility)

☐☐ – ☐☐ – ☐☐☐☐
Month   Day   Year

A1700. Type of Entry

Enter Code ☐
1. Admission
2. Reentry

A1800. Entered From

Enter Code ☐☐
01. **Community** (private home/apt., board/care, assisted living, group home)
02. **Another nursing home or swing bed**
03. **Acute hospital**
04. **Psychiatric hospital**
05. **Inpatient rehabilitation facility**
06. **MR/DD facility**
07. **Hospice**
09. **Long Term Care Hospital** (LTCH)
99. **Other**

A2000. Discharge Date

Complete only if A0310F = 10, 11, or 12

☐☐ – ☐☐ – ☐☐☐☐
Month   Day   Year

A2100. Discharge Status

Complete only if A0310F = 10, 11, or 12

Enter Code ☐☐
01. **Community** (private home/apt., board/care, assisted living, group home)
02. **Another nursing home or swing bed**
03. **Acute hospital**
04. **Psychiatric hospital**
05. **Inpatient rehabilitation facility**
06. **MR/DD facility**
07. **Hospice**
08. **Deceased**
09. **Long Term Care Hospital** (LTCH)
99. **Other**

Section A — Identification Information

A2200. Previous Assessment Reference Date for Significant Correction
Complete only if A0310A = 05 or 06

☐ ☐ – ☐ ☐ – ☐ ☐ ☐ ☐		
Month	Day	Year

A2300. Assessment Reference Date

Observation end date:

☐ ☐ – ☐ ☐ – ☐ ☐ ☐ ☐		
Month	Day	Year

A2400. Medicare Stay

Enter Code ☐

A. Has the resident had a Medicare-covered stay since the most recent entry?

   0. **No** → Skip to B0100, Comatose
   1. **Yes** → Continue to A2400B, Start date of most recent Medicare stay

B. Start date of most recent Medicare stay:

☐ ☐ – ☐ ☐ – ☐ ☐ ☐ ☐		
Month	Day	Year

C. End date of most recent Medicare stay - Enter dashes if stay is ongoing:

☐ ☐ – ☐ ☐ – ☐ ☐ ☐ ☐		
Month	Day	Year

Look back period for all items is 7 days unless another time frame is indicated

Section B	Hearing, Speech, and Vision

B0100. Comatose

Enter Code	**Persistent vegetative state/no discernible consciousness** 0. **No** → Continue to B0200, Hearing 1. **Yes** → Skip to G0110, Activities of Daily Living (ADL) Assistance

B0200. Hearing

Enter Code	**Ability to hear** (with hearing aid or hearing appliances if normally used) 0. **Adequate** - no difficulty in normal conversation, social interaction, listening to TV 1. **Minimal difficulty** - difficulty in some environments (e.g., when person speaks softly or setting is noisy) 2. **Moderate difficulty** - speaker has to increase volume and speak distinctly 3. **Highly impaired** - absence of useful hearing

B0300. Hearing Aid

Enter Code	**Hearing aid or other hearing appliance used** in completing B0200, Hearing 0. **No** 1. **Yes**

B0600. Speech Clarity

Enter Code	**Select best description of speech pattern** 0. **Clear speech** - distinct intelligible words 1. **Unclear speech** - slurred or mumbled words 2. **No speech** - absence of spoken words

B0700. Makes Self Understood

Enter Code	**Ability to express ideas and wants,** consider both verbal and non-verbal expression 0. **Understood** 1. **Usually understood** - difficulty communicating some words or finishing thoughts **but** is able if prompted or given time 2. **Sometimes understood** - ability is limited to making concrete requests 3. **Rarely/never understood**

B0800. Ability To Understand Others

Enter Code	**Understanding verbal content, however able** (with hearing aid or device if used) 0. **Understands** - clear comprehension 1. **Usually understands** - misses some part/intent of message **but** comprehends most conversation 2. **Sometimes understands** - responds adequately to simple, direct communication only 3. **Rarely/never understands**

B1000. Vision

Enter Code	**Ability to see in adequate light** (with glasses or other visual appliances) 0. **Adequate** - sees fine detail, such as regular print in newspapers/books 1. **Impaired** - sees large print, but not regular print in newspapers/books 2. **Moderately impaired** - limited vision; not able to see newspaper headlines but can identify objects 3. **Highly impaired** - object identification in question, but eyes appear to follow objects 4. **Severely impaired** - no vision or sees only light, colors or shapes; eyes do not appear to follow objects

B1200. Corrective Lenses

Enter Code	**Corrective lenses (contacts, glasses, or magnifying glass) used** in completing B1000, Vision 0. **No** 1. **Yes**

Section C — Cognitive Patterns

C0100. Should Brief Interview for Mental Status (C0200-C0500) be Conducted?
Attempt to conduct interview with all residents

Enter Code [ ]
    0. **No** (resident is rarely/never understood) → Skip to and complete C0700-C1000, Staff Assessment for Mental Status
    1. **Yes** → Continue to C0200, Repetition of Three Words

---

Brief Interview for Mental Status (BIMS)

C0200. Repetition of Three Words

Enter Code [ ]
Ask resident: *"I am going to say three words for you to remember. Please repeat the words after I have said all three. The words are: **sock, blue, and bed.** Now tell me the three words."*
Number of words repeated after first attempt
    0. **None**
    1. **One**
    2. **Two**
    3. **Three**
After the resident's first attempt, repeat the words using cues ("*sock, something to wear; blue, a color; bed, a piece of furniture*"). You may repeat the words up to two more times.

C0300. Temporal Orientation (orientation to year, month, and day)

Enter Code [ ]
Ask resident: *"Please tell me what year it is right now."*
A. Able to report correct year
    0. **Missed by > 5 years** or no answer
    1. **Missed by 2-5 years**
    2. **Missed by 1 year**
    3. **Correct**

Enter Code [ ]
Ask resident: *"What month are we in right now?"*
B. Able to report correct month
    0. **Missed by > 1 month** or no answer
    1. **Missed by 6 days to 1 month**
    2. **Accurate within 5 days**

Enter Code [ ]
Ask resident: *"What day of the week is today?"*
C. Able to report correct day of the week
    0. **Incorrect** or no answer
    1. **Correct**

C0400. Recall

Enter Code [ ]
Ask resident: *"Let's go back to an earlier question. What were those three words that I asked you to repeat?"*
If unable to remember a word, give cue (something to wear; a color; a piece of furniture) for that word.
A. Able to recall "sock"
    0. **No** - could not recall
    1. **Yes, after cueing** ("something to wear")
    2. **Yes, no cue required**

Enter Code [ ]
B. Able to recall "blue"
    0. **No** - could not recall
    1. **Yes, after cueing** ("a color")
    2. **Yes, no cue required**

Enter Code [ ]
C. Able to recall "bed"
    0. **No** - could not recall
    1. **Yes, after cueing** ("a piece of furniture")
    2. **Yes, no cue required**

C0500. Summary Score

Enter Score [ ][ ]
Add scores for questions C0200-C0400 and fill in total score (00-15)
Enter 99 if the resident was unable to complete the interview

Section C	Cognitive Patterns

C0600. Should the Staff Assessment for Mental Status (C0700 - C1000) be Conducted?

Enter Code [ ]	0. **No** (resident was able to complete interview) → Skip to C1300, Signs and Symptoms of Delirium 1. **Yes** (resident was unable to complete interview) → Continue to C0700, Short-term Memory OK

Staff Assessment for Mental Status

Do not conduct if Brief Interview for Mental Status (C0200-C0500) was completed

C0700. Short-term Memory OK

Enter Code [ ]	**Seems or appears to recall after 5 minutes** 0. **Memory OK** 1. **Memory problem**

C0800. Long-term Memory OK

Enter Code [ ]	**Seems or appears to recall long past** 0. **Memory OK** 1. **Memory problem**

C0900. Memory/Recall Ability

↓ **Check all that the resident was normally able to recall**

[ ]	A. **Current season**
[ ]	B. **Location of own room**
[ ]	C. **Staff names and faces**
[ ]	D. **That he or she is in a nursing home**
[ ]	Z. **None of the above** were recalled

C1000. Cognitive Skills for Daily Decision Making

Enter Code [ ]	**Made decisions regarding tasks of daily life** 0. **Independent** - decisions consistent/reasonable 1. **Modified independence** - some difficulty in new situations only 2. **Moderately impaired** - decisions poor; cues/supervision required 3. **Severely impaired** - never/rarely made decisions

---

Delirium

C1300. Signs and Symptoms of Delirium (from CAM©)

Code **after completing** Brief Interview for Mental Status or Staff Assessment, and reviewing medical record

Coding: 0. **Behavior not present** 1. **Behavior continuously present, does not fluctuate** 2. **Behavior present, fluctuates** (comes and goes, changes in severity)	↓ **Enter Codes in Boxes**	
	[ ]	A. **Inattention** - Did the resident have difficulty focusing attention (easily distracted, out of touch or difficulty following what was said)?
	[ ]	B. **Disorganized thinking** - Was the resident's thinking disorganized or incoherent (rambling or irrelevant conversation, unclear or illogical flow of ideas, or unpredictable switching from subject to subject)?
	[ ]	C. **Altered level of consciousness** - Did the resident have altered level of consciousness (e.g., **vigilant** - startled easily to any sound or touch; **lethargic** - repeatedly dozed off when being asked questions, but responded to voice or touch; **stuporous** - very difficult to arouse and keep aroused for the interview; **comatose** - could not be aroused)?
	[ ]	D. **Psychomotor retardation**- Did the resident have an unusually decreased level of activity such as sluggishness, staring into space, staying in one position, moving very slowly?

C1600. Acute Onset Mental Status Change

Enter Code [ ]	**Is there evidence of an acute change in mental status** from the resident's baseline? 0. **No** 1. **Yes**

MDS 3.0 Nursing Home Comprehensive (NC) Version 1.10.3 Effective 04/01/2012   Page 8 of 40

Section D   Mood

D0100. Should Resident Mood Interview be Conducted? - Attempt to conduct interview with all residents

Enter Code ☐
- 0. **No** (resident is rarely/never understood) → Skip to and complete D0500-D0600, Staff Assessment of Resident Mood (PHQ-9-OV)
- 1. **Yes** → Continue to D0200, Resident Mood Interview (PHQ-9©)

D0200. Resident Mood Interview (PHQ-9©)

Say to resident: *"Over the last 2 weeks, have you been bothered by any of the following problems?"*

If symptom is present, enter 1 (yes) in column 1, Symptom Presence.
If yes in column 1, then ask the resident: "About **how often** have you been bothered by this?"
Read and show the resident a card with the symptom frequency choices. Indicate response in column 2, Symptom Frequency.

1. Symptom Presence
- 0. **No** (enter 0 in column 2)
- 1. **Yes** (enter 0-3 in column 2)
- 9. **No response** (leave column 2 blank)

2. Symptom Frequency
- 0. **Never or 1 day**
- 1. **2-6 days** (several days)
- 2. **7-11 days** (half or more of the days)
- 3. **12-14 days** (nearly every day)

	1. Symptom Presence	2. Symptom Frequency
A. Little interest or pleasure in doing things	☐	☐
B. Feeling down, depressed, or hopeless	☐	☐
C. Trouble falling or staying asleep, or sleeping too much	☐	☐
D. Feeling tired or having little energy	☐	☐
E. Poor appetite or overeating	☐	☐
F. Feeling bad about yourself - or that you are a failure or have let yourself or your family down	☐	☐
G. Trouble concentrating on things, such as reading the newspaper or watching television	☐	☐
H. Moving or speaking so slowly that other people could have noticed. Or the opposite - being so fidgety or restless that you have been moving around a lot more than usual	☐	☐
I. Thoughts that you would be better off dead, or of hurting yourself in some way	☐	☐

D0300. Total Severity Score

☐☐ Add scores for all frequency responses in Column 2, Symptom Frequency. Total score must be between 00 and 27. Enter 99 if unable to complete interview (i.e., Symptom Frequency is blank for 3 or more items).

D0350. Safety Notification - Complete only if D0200I1 = 1 indicating possibility of resident self harm

Enter Code ☐ **Was responsible staff or provider informed that there is a potential for resident self harm?**
- 0. **No**
- 1. **Yes**

MDS 3.0 Nursing Home Comprehensive (NC) Version 1.10.3 Effective 04/01/2012

Section D	Mood

D0500. Staff Assessment of Resident Mood (PHQ-9-OV*)
Do not conduct if Resident Mood Interview (D0200-D0300) was completed

Over the last 2 weeks, did the resident have any of the following problems or behaviors?

If symptom is present, enter 1 (yes) in column 1, Symptom Presence.
Then move to column 2, Symptom Frequency, and indicate symptom frequency.

1. Symptom Presence 0. **No** (enter 0 in column 2) 1. **Yes** (enter 0-3 in column 2)	**2. Symptom Frequency** 0. **Never or 1 day** 1. **2-6 days** (several days) 2. **7-11 days** (half or more of the days) 3. **12-14 days** (nearly every day)	**1.** Symptom Presence	**2.** Symptom Frequency
		↓ Enter Scores in Boxes ↓	
A. Little interest or pleasure in doing things		☐	☐
B. Feeling or appearing down, depressed, or hopeless		☐	☐
C. Trouble falling or staying asleep, or sleeping too much		☐	☐
D. Feeling tired or having little energy		☐	☐
E. Poor appetite or overeating		☐	☐
F. Indicating that s/he feels bad about self, is a failure, or has let self or family down		☐	☐
G. Trouble concentrating on things, such as reading the newspaper or watching television		☐	☐
H. Moving or speaking so slowly that other people have noticed. Or the opposite - being so fidgety or restless that s/he has been moving around a lot more than usual		☐	☐
I. States that life isn't worth living, wishes for death, or attempts to harm self		☐	☐
J. Being short-tempered, easily annoyed		☐	☐

D0600. Total Severity Score

☐☐ **Add scores for all frequency responses in Column 2**, Symptom Frequency. Total score must be between 00 and 30.
Enter Score

D0650. Safety Notification - Complete only if D0500I1 = 1 indicating possibility of resident self harm

Enter Code **Was responsible staff or provider informed that there is a potential for resident self harm?**
☐   0. **No**
           1. **Yes**

Section E	Behavior

E0100. Potential Indicators of Psychosis

↓ Check all that apply

☐	**A. Hallucinations** (perceptual experiences in the absence of real external sensory stimuli)
☐	**B. Delusions** (misconceptions or beliefs that are firmly held, contrary to reality)
☐	**Z. None of the above**

Behavioral Symptoms

E0200. Behavioral Symptom - Presence & Frequency

Note presence of symptoms and their frequency

	↓ Enter Codes in Boxes
Coding: 0. **Behavior not exhibited** 1. **Behavior of this type occurred 1 to 3 days** 2. **Behavior of this type occurred 4 to 6 days,** but less than daily 3. **Behavior of this type occurred daily**	☐ **A.** **Physical behavioral symptoms directed toward others** (e.g., hitting, kicking, pushing, scratching, grabbing, abusing others sexually)
	☐ **B.** **Verbal behavioral symptoms directed toward others** (e.g., threatening others, screaming at others, cursing at others)
	☐ **C.** **Other behavioral symptoms not directed toward others** (e.g., physical symptoms such as hitting or scratching self, pacing, rummaging, public sexual acts, disrobing in public, throwing or smearing food or bodily wastes, or verbal/vocal symptoms like screaming, disruptive sounds)

E0300. Overall Presence of Behavioral Symptoms

Enter Code ☐	Were any behavioral symptoms in questions E0200 coded 1, 2, or 3? 0. **No** → Skip to E0800, Rejection of Care 1. **Yes** → Considering all of E0200, Behavioral Symptoms, answer E0500 and E0600 below

E0500. Impact on Resident

	Did any of the identified symptom(s):
Enter Code ☐	**A. Put the resident at significant risk for physical illness or injury?** 0. **No** 1. **Yes**
Enter Code ☐	**B. Significantly interfere with the resident's care?** 0. **No** 1. **Yes**
Enter Code ☐	**C. Significantly interfere with the resident's participation in activities or social interactions?** 0. **No** 1. **Yes**

E0600. Impact on Others

	Did any of the identified symptom(s):
Enter Code ☐	**A. Put others at significant risk for physical injury?** 0. **No** 1. **Yes**
Enter Code ☐	**B. Significantly intrude on the privacy or activity of others?** 0. **No** 1. **Yes**
Enter Code ☐	**C. Significantly disrupt care or living environment?** 0. **No** 1. **Yes**

E0800. Rejection of Care - Presence & Frequency

Enter Code ☐	Did the resident reject evaluation or care (e.g., bloodwork, taking medications, ADL assistance) **that is necessary to achieve the resident's goals for health and well-being?** Do not include behaviors that have already been addressed (e.g., by discussion or care planning with the resident or family), and determined to be consistent with resident values, preferences, or goals. 0. **Behavior not exhibited** 1. **Behavior of this type occurred 1 to 3 days** 2. **Behavior of this type occurred 4 to 6 days,** but less than daily 3. **Behavior of this type occurred daily**

MDS 3.0 Nursing Home Comprehensive (NC) Version 1.10.3 Effective 04/01/2012   Page 11 of 40

Section E	Behavior

E0900. Wandering - Presence & Frequency

Enter Code	**Has the resident wandered?** 0. **Behavior not exhibited** → Skip to E1100, Change in Behavioral or Other Symptoms 1. **Behavior of this type occurred 1 to 3 days** 2. **Behavior of this type occurred 4 to 6 days**, but less than daily 3. **Behavior of this type occurred daily**

E1000. Wandering - Impact

Enter Code	**A. Does the wandering place the resident at significant risk of getting to a potentially dangerous place** (e.g., stairs, outside of the facility)? 0. **No** 1. **Yes**
Enter Code	**B. Does the wandering significantly intrude on the privacy or activities of others?** 0. **No** 1. **Yes**

E1100. Change in Behavior or Other Symptoms

Consider all of the symptoms assessed in items E0100 through E1000

Enter Code	How does resident's current behavior status, care rejection, or wandering **compare to prior assessment (OBRA or Scheduled PPS)?** 0. **Same** 1. **Improved** 2. **Worse** 3. **N/A** because no prior MDS assessment

Section F	Preferences for Customary Routine and Activities

F0300. Should Interview for Daily and Activity Preferences be Conducted? - Attempt to interview all residents able to communicate. If resident is unable to complete, attempt to complete interview with family member or significant other

Enter Code
☐

   0. **No** (resident is rarely/never understood <u>and</u> family/significant other not available) → Skip to and complete F0800, Staff Assessment of Daily and Activity Preferences
   1. **Yes** → Continue to F0400, Interview for Daily Preferences

---

F0400. Interview for Daily Preferences

Show resident the response options and say: **"While you are in this facility..."**

↓ Enter Codes in Boxes

Coding:
1. **Very important**
2. **Somewhat important**
3. **Not very important**
4. **Not important at all**
5. **Important, but can't do or no choice**
9. **No response or non-responsive**

☐ A. *how important is it to you to* **choose what clothes to wear?**

☐ B. *how important is it to you to* **take care of your personal belongings or things?**

☐ C. *how important is it to you to* **choose between a tub bath, shower, bed bath, or sponge bath?**

☐ D. *how important is it to you to* **have snacks available between meals?**

☐ E. *how important is it to you to* **choose your own bedtime?**

☐ F. *how important is it to you to* **have your family or a close friend involved in discussions about your care?**

☐ G. *how important is it to you to* **be able to use the phone in private?**

☐ H. *how important is it to you to* **have a place to lock your things to keep them safe?**

F0500. Interview for Activity Preferences

Show resident the response options and say: **"While you are in this facility..."**

↓ Enter Codes in Boxes

Coding:
1. **Very important**
2. **Somewhat important**
3. **Not very important**
4. **Not important at all**
5. **Important, but can't do or no choice**
9. **No response or non-responsive**

☐ A. *how important is it to you to* **have books, newspapers, and magazines to read?**

☐ B. *how important is it to you to* **listen to music you like?**

☐ C. *how important is it to you to* **be around animals such as pets?**

☐ D. *how important is it to you to* **keep up with the news?**

☐ E. *how important is it to you to* **do things with groups of people?**

☐ F. *how important is it to you to* **do your favorite activities?**

☐ G. *how important is it to you to* **go outside to get fresh air when the weather is good?**

☐ H. *how important is it to you to* **participate in religious services or practices?**

F0600. Daily and Activity Preferences Primary Respondent

Enter Code
☐

Indicate primary respondent for Daily and Activity Preferences (F0400 and F0500)
   1. **Resident**
   2. **Family or significant other** (close friend or other representative)
   9. **Interview could not be completed** by resident or family/significant other ("No response" to 3 or more items")

MDS 3.0 Nursing Home Comprehensive (NC) Version 1.10.3 Effective 04/01/2012

Page 13 of 40

Section F	Preferences for Customary Routine and Activities

F0700. Should the Staff Assessment of Daily and Activity Preferences be Conducted?

Enter Code
☐

0. **No** (because Interview for Daily and Activity Preferences (F0400 and F0500) was completed by resident or family/significant other) → Skip to and complete G0110, Activities of Daily Living (ADL) Assistance

1. **Yes** (because 3 or more items in Interview for Daily and Activity Preferences (F0400 and F0500) were not completed by resident or family/significant other) → Continue to F0800, Staff Assessment of Daily and Activity Preferences

F0800. Staff Assessment of Daily and Activity Preferences

Do not conduct if Interview for Daily and Activity Preferences (F0400-F0500) was completed

Resident Prefers:

↓ Check all that apply

☐	A. Choosing clothes to wear
☐	B. Caring for personal belongings
☐	C. Receiving tub bath
☐	D. Receiving shower
☐	E. Receiving bed bath
☐	F. Receiving sponge bath
☐	G. Snacks between meals
☐	H. Staying up past 8:00 p.m.
☐	I. Family or significant other involvement in care discussions
☐	J. Use of phone in private
☐	K. Place to lock personal belongings
☐	L. Reading books, newspapers, or magazines
☐	M. Listening to music
☐	N. Being around animals such as pets
☐	O. Keeping up with the news
☐	P. Doing things with groups of people
☐	Q. Participating in favorite activities
☐	R. Spending time away from the nursing home
☐	S. Spending time outdoors
☐	T. Participating in religious activities or practices
☐	Z. None of the above

For Activity Programs   **171**

Resident _____   Identifier _____   Date _____

Section G	Functional Status

G0110. Activities of Daily Living (ADL) Assistance
Refer to the ADL flow chart in the RAI manual to facilitate accurate coding

Instructions for Rule of 3
- When an activity occurs three times at any one given level, code that level.
- When an activity occurs three times at multiple levels, code the most dependent, exceptions are total dependence (4), activity must require full assist every time, and activity did not occur (8), activity must not have occurred at all. Example, three times extensive assistance (3) and three times limited assistance (2), code extensive assistance (3).
- When an activity occurs at various levels, but not three times at any given level, apply the following:
  - When there is a combination of full staff performance, and extensive assistance, code extensive assistance.
  - When there is a combination of full staff performance, weight bearing assistance and/or non-weight bearing assistance code limited assistance (2).

If none of the above are met, code supervision.

1. ADL Self-Performance
Code for **resident's performance** over all shifts - not including setup. If the ADL activity occurred 3 or more times at various levels of assistance, code the most dependent - except for total dependence, which requires full staff performance every time

Coding:

Activity Occurred 3 or More Times
- 0. **Independent** - no help or staff oversight at any time
- 1. **Supervision** - oversight, encouragement or cueing
- 2. **Limited assistance** - resident highly involved in activity; staff provide guided maneuvering of limbs or other non-weight-bearing assistance
- 3. **Extensive assistance** - resident involved in activity, staff provide weight-bearing support
- 4. **Total dependence** - full staff performance every time during entire 7-day period

Activity Occurred 2 or Fewer Times
- 7. **Activity occurred only once or twice** - activity did occur but only once or twice
- 8. **Activity did not occur** - activity did not occur or family and/or non-facility staff provided care 100% of the time for that activity over the entire 7-day period

2. ADL Support Provided
Code for **most support provided** over all shifts; code regardless of resident's self-performance classification

Coding:
- 0. **No** setup or physical help from staff
- 1. **Setup** help only
- 2. **One** person physical assist
- 3. **Two+** persons physical assist
- 8. ADL activity itself **did not occur** or family and/or non-facility staff provided care 100% of the time for that activity over the entire 7-day period

	1. Self-Performance	2. Support
	↓ Enter Codes in Boxes ↓	
A. **Bed mobility** - how resident moves to and from lying position, turns side to side, and positions body while in bed or alternate sleep furniture	☐	☐
B. **Transfer** - how resident moves between surfaces including to or from: bed, chair, wheelchair, standing position (**excludes** to/from bath/toilet)	☐	☐
C. **Walk in room** - how resident walks between locations in his/her room	☐	☐
D. **Walk in corridor** - how resident walks in corridor on unit	☐	☐
E. **Locomotion on unit** - how resident moves between locations in his/her room and adjacent corridor on same floor. If in wheelchair, self-sufficiency once in chair	☐	☐
F. **Locomotion off unit** - how resident moves to and returns from off-unit locations (e.g., areas set aside for dining, activities or treatments). **If facility has only one floor**, how resident moves to and from distant areas on the floor. If in wheelchair, self-sufficiency once in chair	☐	☐
G. **Dressing** - how resident puts on, fastens and takes off all items of clothing, including donning/removing a prosthesis or TED hose. Dressing includes putting on and changing pajamas and housedresses	☐	☐
H. **Eating** - how resident eats and drinks, regardless of skill. Do not include eating/drinking during medication pass. Includes intake of nourishment by other means (e.g., tube feeding, total parenteral nutrition, IV fluids administered for nutrition or hydration)	☐	☐
I. **Toilet use** - how resident uses the toilet room, commode, bedpan, or urinal; transfers on/off toilet; cleanses self after elimination; changes pad; manages ostomy or catheter; and adjusts clothes. Do not include emptying of bedpan, urinal, bedside commode, catheter bag or ostomy bag	☐	☐
J. **Personal hygiene** - how resident maintains personal hygiene, including combing hair, brushing teeth, shaving, applying makeup, washing/drying face and hands (**excludes** baths and showers)	☐	☐

Section G   Functional Status

G0120. Bathing

How resident takes full-body bath/shower, sponge bath, and transfers in/out of tub/shower (**excludes** washing of back and hair). Code for **most dependent** in self-performance and support

Enter Code	A. Self-performance
☐	0. **Independent** - no help provided 1. **Supervision** - oversight help only 2. **Physical help limited to transfer only** 3. **Physical help in part of bathing activity** 4. **Total dependence** 8. **Activity itself did not occur** or family and/or non-facility staff provided care 100% of the time for that activity over the entire 7-day period
Enter Code ☐	B. **Support provided** (Bathing support codes are as defined in item **G0110 column 2, ADL Support Provided**, above)

G0300. Balance During Transitions and Walking

After observing the resident, **code the following walking and transition items for most dependent**

Coding:	↓ Enter Codes in Boxes	
0. **Steady at all times** 1. **Not steady, but <u>able</u> to stabilize without staff assistance** 2. **Not steady, <u>only able</u> to stabilize with staff assistance** 8. **Activity did not occur**	☐	A. **Moving from seated to standing position**
	☐	B. **Walking** (with assistive device if used)
	☐	C. **Turning around** and facing the opposite direction while walking
	☐	D. **Moving on and off toilet**
	☐	E. **Surface-to-surface transfer** (transfer between bed and chair or wheelchair)

G0400. Functional Limitation in Range of Motion

Code for limitation that interfered with daily functions or placed resident at risk of injury

Coding:	↓ Enter Codes in Boxes	
0. **No impairment** 1. **Impairment on one side** 2. **Impairment on both sides**	☐	A. **Upper extremity** (shoulder, elbow, wrist, hand)
	☐	B. **Lower extremity** (hip, knee, ankle, foot)

G0600. Mobility Devices

↓ **Check all that were normally used**

☐	A. **Cane/crutch**
☐	B. **Walker**
☐	C. **Wheelchair** (manual or electric)
☐	D. **Limb prosthesis**
☐	Z. **None of the above** were used

G0900. Functional Rehabilitation Potential
Complete only if A0310A = 01

Enter Code ☐	A. **Resident believes he or she is capable of increased independence** in at least some ADLs 0. **No** 1. **Yes** 9. **Unable to determine**
Enter Code ☐	B. **Direct care staff believe resident is capable of increased independence** in at least some ADLs 0. **No** 1. **Yes**

Section H	Bladder and Bowel

H0100. Appliances

↓ Check all that apply

☐	**A. Indwelling catheter** (including suprapubic catheter and nephrostomy tube)
☐	**B. External catheter**
☐	**C. Ostomy** (including urostomy, ileostomy, and colostomy)
☐	**D. Intermittent catheterization**
☐	**Z. None of the above**

H0200. Urinary Toileting Program

Enter Code ☐	**A. Has a trial of a toileting program (e.g., scheduled toileting, prompted voiding, or bladder training)** been attempted on admission/entry or reentry or since urinary incontinence was noted in this facility?
	  0. **No** → Skip to H0300, Urinary Continence
	  1. **Yes** → Continue to H0200B, Response
	  9. **Unable to determine** → Skip to H0200C, Current toileting program or trial

Enter Code ☐	**B. Response** - What was the resident's response to the trial program?
	  0. **No improvement**
	  1. **Decreased wetness**
	  2. **Completely dry** (continent)
	  9. **Unable to determine** or trial in progress

Enter Code ☐	**C. Current toileting program or trial** - Is a toileting program (e.g., scheduled toileting, prompted voiding, or bladder training) currently being used to manage the resident's urinary continence?
	  0. **No**
	  1. **Yes**

H0300. Urinary Continence

Enter Code ☐	**Urinary continence** - Select the one category that best describes the resident
	  0. **Always continent**
	  1. **Occasionally incontinent** (less than 7 episodes of incontinence)
	  2. **Frequently incontinent** (7 or more episodes of urinary incontinence, but at least one episode of continent voiding)
	  3. **Always incontinent** (no episodes of continent voiding)
	  9. **Not rated,** resident had a catheter (indwelling, condom), urinary ostomy, or no urine output for the entire 7 days

H0400. Bowel Continence

Enter Code ☐	**Bowel continence** - Select the one category that best describes the resident
	  0. **Always continent**
	  1. **Occasionally incontinent** (one episode of bowel incontinence)
	  2. **Frequently incontinent** (2 or more episodes of bowel incontinence, but at least one continent bowel movement)
	  3. **Always incontinent** (no episodes of continent bowel movements)
	  9. **Not rated,** resident had an ostomy or did not have a bowel movement for the entire 7 days

H0500. Bowel Toileting Program

Enter Code ☐	**Is a toileting program currently being used to manage the resident's bowel continence?**
	  0. **No**
	  1. **Yes**

H0600. Bowel Patterns

Enter Code ☐	**Constipation present?**
	  0. **No**
	  1. **Yes**

Section I	Active Diagnoses

Active Diagnoses in the last 7 days - Check all that apply
Diagnoses listed in parentheses are provided as examples and should not be considered as all-inclusive lists

Cancer
- [ ] **I0100. Cancer** (with or without metastasis)

Heart/Circulation
- [ ] **I0200. Anemia** (e.g., aplastic, iron deficiency, pernicious, and sickle cell)
- [ ] **I0300. Atrial Fibrillation or Other Dysrhythmias** (e.g., bradycardias and tachycardias)
- [ ] **I0400. Coronary Artery Disease (CAD)** (e.g., angina, myocardial infarction, and atherosclerotic heart disease (ASHD))
- [ ] **I0500. Deep Venous Thrombosis (DVT), Pulmonary Embolus (PE), or Pulmonary Thrombo-Embolism (PTE)**
- [ ] **I0600. Heart Failure** (e.g., congestive heart failure (CHF) and pulmonary edema)
- [ ] **I0700. Hypertension**
- [ ] **I0800. Orthostatic Hypotension**
- [ ] **I0900. Peripheral Vascular Disease (PVD) or Peripheral Arterial Disease (PAD)**

Gastrointestinal
- [ ] **I1100. Cirrhosis**
- [ ] **I1200. Gastroesophageal Reflux Disease (GERD) or Ulcer** (e.g., esophageal, gastric, and peptic ulcers)
- [ ] **I1300. Ulcerative Colitis, Crohn's Disease, or Inflammatory Bowel Disease**

Genitourinary
- [ ] **I1400. Benign Prostatic Hyperplasia (BPH)**
- [ ] **I1500. Renal Insufficiency, Renal Failure, or End-Stage Renal Disease (ESRD)**
- [ ] **I1550. Neurogenic Bladder**
- [ ] **I1650. Obstructive Uropathy**

Infections
- [ ] **I1700. Multidrug-Resistant Organism (MDRO)**
- [ ] **I2000. Pneumonia**
- [ ] **I2100. Septicemia**
- [ ] **I2200. Tuberculosis**
- [ ] **I2300. Urinary Tract Infection (UTI) (LAST 30 DAYS)**
- [ ] **I2400. Viral Hepatitis** (e.g., Hepatitis A, B, C, D, and E)
- [ ] **I2500. Wound Infection** (other than foot)

Metabolic
- [ ] **I2900. Diabetes Mellitus (DM)** (e.g., diabetic retinopathy, nephropathy, and neuropathy)
- [ ] **I3100. Hyponatremia**
- [ ] **I3200. Hyperkalemia**
- [ ] **I3300. Hyperlipidemia** (e.g., hypercholesterolemia)
- [ ] **I3400. Thyroid Disorder** (e.g., hypothyroidism, hyperthyroidism, and Hashimoto's thyroiditis)

Musculoskeletal
- [ ] **I3700. Arthritis** (e.g., degenerative joint disease (DJD), osteoarthritis, and rheumatoid arthritis (RA))
- [ ] **I3800. Osteoporosis**
- [ ] **I3900. Hip Fracture** - any hip fracture that has a relationship to current status, treatments, monitoring (e.g., sub-capital fractures, and fractures of the trochanter and femoral neck)
- [ ] **I4000. Other Fracture**

Neurological
- [ ] **I4200. Alzheimer's Disease**
- [ ] **I4300. Aphasia**
- [ ] **I4400. Cerebral Palsy**
- [ ] **I4500. Cerebrovascular Accident (CVA), Transient Ischemic Attack (TIA), or Stroke**
- [ ] **I4800. Non-Alzheimer's Dementia** (e.g. Lewy body dementia, vascular or multi-infarct dementia; mixed dementia; frontotemporal dementia such as Pick's disease; and dementia related to stroke, Parkinson's or Creutzfeldt-Jakob diseases)

Neurological Diagnoses continued on next page

MDS 3.0 Nursing Home Comprehensive (NC) Version 1.10.3 Effective 04/01/2012 Page 18 of 40

Section I	Active Diagnoses

Active Diagnoses in the last 7 days - Check all that apply
Diagnoses listed in parentheses are provided as examples and should not be considered as all-inclusive lists

Neurological - Continued

☐ I4900. **Hemiplegia or Hemiparesis**

☐ I5000. **Paraplegia**

☐ I5100. **Quadriplegia**

☐ I5200. **Multiple Sclerosis (MS)**

☐ I5250. **Huntington's Disease**

☐ I5300. **Parkinson's Disease**

☐ I5350. **Tourette's Syndrome**

☐ I5400. **Seizure Disorder or Epilepsy**

☐ I5500. **Traumatic Brain Injury (TBI)**

Nutritional

☐ I5600. **Malnutrition** (protein or calorie) or at risk for malnutrition

Psychiatric/Mood Disorder

☐ I5700. **Anxiety Disorder**

☐ I5800. **Depression** (other than bipolar)

☐ I5900. **Manic Depression** (bipolar disease)

☐ I5950. **Psychotic Disorder** (other than schizophrenia)

☐ I6000. **Schizophrenia** (e.g., schizoaffective and schizophreniform disorders)

☐ I6100. **Post Traumatic Stress Disorder (PTSD)**

Pulmonary

☐ I6200. **Asthma, Chronic Obstructive Pulmonary Disease (COPD), or Chronic Lung Disease** (e.g., chronic bronchitis and restrictive lung diseases such as asbestosis)

☐ I6300. **Respiratory Failure**

Vision

☐ I6500. **Cataracts, Glaucoma, or Macular Degeneration**

None of Above

☐ I7900. **None of the above active diagnoses** within the last 7 days

Other

I8000. Additional active diagnoses
Enter diagnosis on line and ICD code in boxes. Include the decimal for the code in the appropriate box.

A. _____ ☐☐☐☐☐ ☐☐☐

B. _____ ☐☐☐☐☐ ☐☐☐

C. _____ ☐☐☐☐☐ ☐☐☐

D. _____ ☐☐☐☐☐ ☐☐☐

E. _____ ☐☐☐☐☐ ☐☐☐

F. _____ ☐☐☐☐☐ ☐☐☐

G. _____ ☐☐☐☐☐ ☐☐☐

H. _____ ☐☐☐☐☐ ☐☐☐

I. _____ ☐☐☐☐☐ ☐☐☐

J. _____ ☐☐☐☐☐ ☐☐☐

Section J   Health Conditions

J0100. Pain Management - Complete for all residents, regardless of current pain level

At any time in the last **5** days, has the resident:

Enter Code	
☐	**A. Received scheduled pain medication regimen?** 0. **No** 1. **Yes**
☐	**B. Received PRN pain medications OR was offered and declined?** 0. **No** 1. **Yes**
☐	**C. Received non-medication intervention for pain?** 0. **No** 1. **Yes**

J0200. Should Pain Assessment Interview be Conducted?
Attempt to conduct interview with all residents. If resident is comatose, skip to J1100, Shortness of Breath (dyspnea)

Enter Code	
☐	0. **No** (resident is rarely/never understood) → Skip to and complete J0800, Indicators of Pain or Possible Pain 1. **Yes** → Continue to J0300, Pain Presence

Pain Assessment Interview

J0300. Pain Presence

Enter Code	
☐	Ask resident: "**Have you had pain or hurting at any time** in the last 5 days?" 0. **No** → Skip to J1100, Shortness of Breath 1. **Yes** → Continue to J0400, Pain Frequency 9. **Unable to answer** → Skip to J0800, Indicators of Pain or Possible Pain

J0400. Pain Frequency

Enter Code	
☐	Ask resident: "**How much of the time have you experienced pain or hurting** over the last 5 days?" 1. **Almost constantly** 2. **Frequently** 3. **Occasionally** 4. **Rarely** 9. **Unable to answer**

J0500. Pain Effect on Function

Enter Code	
☐	**A.** Ask resident: "*Over the past 5 days, **has pain made it hard for you to sleep at night**?*" 0. **No** 1. **Yes** 9. **Unable to answer**
☐	**B.** Ask resident: "*Over the past 5 days, **have you limited your day-to-day activities because of pain**?*" 0. **No** 1. **Yes** 9. **Unable to answer**

J0600. Pain Intensity - Administer **ONLY ONE** of the following pain intensity questions (A or B)

Enter Rating ☐☐	**A. Numeric Rating Scale (00-10)** Ask resident: "*Please rate your worst pain over the last 5 days on a zero to ten scale, with zero being no pain and ten as the worst pain you can imagine.*" (Show resident 00 -10 pain scale) **Enter two-digit response. Enter 99 if unable to answer.**
Enter Code ☐	**B. Verbal Descriptor Scale** Ask resident: "*Please rate the intensity of your worst pain over the last 5 days.*" (Show resident verbal scale) 1. **Mild** 2. **Moderate** 3. **Severe** 4. **Very severe, horrible** 9. **Unable to answer**

MDS 3.0 Nursing Home Comprehensive (NC) Version 1.10.3 Effective 04/01/2012

Section J	Health Conditions

J0700. Should the Staff Assessment for Pain be Conducted?

Enter Code	0. **No** (J0400 = 1 thru 4) → Skip to J1100, Shortness of Breath (dyspnea)
☐	1. **Yes** (J0400 = 9) → Continue to J0800, Indicators of Pain or Possible Pain

Staff Assessment for Pain

J0800. Indicators of Pain or Possible Pain in the last 5 days

↓ **Check all that apply**

☐	A. **Non-verbal sounds** (e.g., crying, whining, gasping, moaning, or groaning)
☐	B. **Vocal complaints of pain** (e.g., that hurts, ouch, stop)
☐	C. **Facial expressions** (e.g., grimaces, winces, wrinkled forehead, furrowed brow, clenched teeth or jaw)
☐	D. **Protective body movements or postures** (e.g., bracing, guarding, rubbing or massaging a body part/area, clutching or holding a body part during movement)
☐	Z. **None of these signs observed or documented** → If checked, skip to J1100, Shortness of Breath (dyspnea)

J0850. Frequency of Indicator of Pain or Possible Pain in the last 5 days

Enter Code	Frequency with which resident complains or shows evidence of pain or possible pain
☐	1. **Indicators of pain** or possible pain observed **1 to 2 days**
	2. **Indicators of pain** or possible pain observed **3 to 4 days**
	3. **Indicators of pain** or possible pain observed **daily**

Other Health Conditions

J1100. Shortness of Breath (dyspnea)

↓ **Check all that apply**

☐	A. **Shortness of breath** or trouble breathing **with exertion** (e.g., walking, bathing, transferring)
☐	B. **Shortness of breath** or trouble breathing **when sitting at rest**
☐	C. **Shortness of breath** or trouble breathing **when lying flat**
☐	Z. **None of the above**

J1300. Current Tobacco Use

Enter Code	Tobacco use
☐	0. **No**
	1. **Yes**

J1400. Prognosis

Enter Code	Does the resident have a condition or chronic disease that may result in a **life expectancy of less than 6 months?** (Requires physician documentation)
☐	0. **No**
	1. **Yes**

J1550. Problem Conditions

↓ **Check all that apply**

☐	A. **Fever**
☐	B. **Vomiting**
☐	C. **Dehydrated**
☐	D. **Internal bleeding**
☐	Z. **None of the above**

MDS 3.0 Nursing Home Comprehensive (NC) Version 1.10.3 Effective 04/01/2012

Section J Health Conditions

J1700. Fall History on Admission/Entry or Reentry
Complete only if A0310A = 01 or A0310E = 1

Enter Code	A.	Did the resident have a fall any time in the **last month** prior to admission/entry or reentry?
☐		0. **No**
		1. **Yes**
		9. **Unable to determine**

Enter Code	B.	Did the resident have a fall any time in the **last 2-6 months** prior to admission/entry or reentry?
☐		0. **No**
		1. **Yes**
		9. **Unable to determine**

Enter Code	C.	Did the resident have any **fracture related to a fall in the 6 months** prior to admission/entry or reentry?
☐		0. **No**
		1. **Yes**
		9. **Unable to determine**

J1800. Any Falls Since Admission/Entry or Reentry or Prior Assessment (OBRA or Scheduled PPS), whichever is more recent

Enter Code	Has the resident **had any falls since admission/entry or reentry or the prior assessment** (OBRA or Scheduled PPS), whichever is more recent?
☐	0. **No** → Skip to K0100, Swallowing Disorder
	1. **Yes** → Continue to J1900, Number of Falls Since Admission/Entry or Reentry or Prior Assessment (OBRA or Scheduled PPS)

J1900. Number of Falls Since Admission/Entry or Reentry or Prior Assessment (OBRA or Scheduled PPS), whichever is more recent

↓ **Enter Codes in Boxes**

Coding:		
0. **None**	☐	A. **No injury** - no evidence of any injury is noted on physical assessment by the nurse or primary care clinician; no complaints of pain or injury by the resident; no change in the resident's behavior is noted after the fall
1. **One**	☐	B. **Injury (except major)** - skin tears, abrasions, lacerations, superficial bruises, hematomas and sprains; or any fall-related injury that causes the resident to complain of pain
2. **Two or more**	☐	C. **Major injury** - bone fractures, joint dislocations, closed head injuries with altered consciousness, subdural hematoma

Section K	Swallowing/Nutritional Status

K0100. Swallowing Disorder

Signs and symptoms of possible swallowing disorder

↓ Check all that apply

- ☐ A. Loss of liquids/solids from mouth when eating or drinking
- ☐ B. Holding food in mouth/cheeks or residual food in mouth after meals
- ☐ C. Coughing or choking during meals or when swallowing medications
- ☐ D. Complaints of difficulty or pain with swallowing
- ☐ Z. None of the above

K0200. Height and Weight - While measuring, if the number is X.1 - X.4 round down; X.5 or greater round up

☐☐ inches
A. Height (in inches). Record most recent height measure since the most recent admission/entry or reentry

☐☐☐ pounds
B. Weight (in pounds). Base weight on most recent measure in last 30 days; measure weight consistently, according to standard facility practice (e.g., in a.m. after voiding, before meal, with shoes off, etc.)

K0300. Weight Loss

Enter Code ☐

Loss of 5% or more in the last month or loss of 10% or more in last 6 months
0. **No** or unknown
1. **Yes, on** physician-prescribed weight-loss regimen
2. **Yes, not on** physician-prescribed weight-loss regimen

K0310. Weight Gain

Enter Code ☐

Gain of 5% or more in the last month or gain of 10% or more in last 6 months
0. **No** or unknown
1. **Yes, on** physician-prescribed weight-gain regimen
2. **Yes, not on** physician-prescribed weight-gain regimen

K0510. Nutritional Approaches

Check all of the following nutritional approaches that were performed during the last **7 days**

	1. While NOT a Resident	2. While a Resident
1. While NOT a Resident Performed *while NOT a resident* of this facility and within the *last 7 days*. Only check column 1 if resident entered (admission or reentry) IN THE LAST 7 DAYS. If resident last entered 7 or more days ago, leave column 1 blank **2. While a Resident** Performed *while a resident* of this facility and within the *last 7 days*	**1. While NOT a Resident**	**2. While a Resident**
	↓ Check all that apply ↓	
A. Parenteral/IV feeding	☐	☐
B. Feeding tube - nasogastric or abdominal (PEG)	☐	☐
C. Mechanically altered diet - require change in texture of food or liquids (e.g., pureed food, thickened liquids)	☐	☐
D. Therapeutic diet (e.g., low salt, diabetic, low cholesterol)	☐	☐
Z. None of the above	☐	☐

K0700. Percent Intake by Artificial Route - Complete K0700 only if K0510A2 or K0510B2 is checked

Enter Code ☐

A. Proportion of total calories the resident received through parenteral or tube feeding
1. **25% or less**
2. **26-50%**
3. **51% or more**

Enter Code ☐

B. Average fluid intake per day by IV or tube feeding
1. **500 cc/day or less**
2. **501 cc/day or more**

Section L	Oral/Dental Status

L0200. Dental

↓ Check all that apply

☐	A. **Broken or loosely fitting full or partial denture** (chipped, cracked, uncleanable, or loose)
☐	B. **No natural teeth or tooth fragment(s)** (edentulous)
☐	C. **Abnormal mouth tissue** (ulcers, masses, oral lesions, including under denture or partial if one is worn)
☐	D. **Obvious or likely cavity or broken natural teeth**
☐	E. **Inflamed or bleeding gums or loose natural teeth**
☐	F. **Mouth or facial pain, discomfort or difficulty with chewing**
☐	G. **Unable to examine**
☐	Z. **None of the above were present**

Section M	Skin Conditions

Report based on highest stage of existing ulcer(s) at its worst; do not "reverse" stage

---

M0100. Determination of Pressure Ulcer Risk

↓ Check all that apply

- [ ] **A.** Resident has a stage 1 or greater, a scar over bony prominence, or a non-removable dressing/device
- [ ] **B.** Formal assessment instrument/tool (e.g., Braden, Norton, or other)
- [ ] **C.** Clinical assessment
- [ ] **Z.** None of the above

M0150. Risk of Pressure Ulcers

Enter Code [ ]
Is this resident at risk of developing pressure ulcers?
0. **No**
1. **Yes**

M0210. Unhealed Pressure Ulcer(s)

Enter Code [ ]
Does this resident have one or more unhealed pressure ulcer(s) at Stage 1 or higher?
0. **No** → Skip to M0900, Healed Pressure Ulcers
1. **Yes** → Continue to M0300, Current Number of Unhealed (non-epithelialized) Pressure Ulcers at Each Stage

---

M0300. Current Number of Unhealed (non-epithelialized) **Pressure Ulcers at Each Stage**

Enter Number [ ]
A. Number of Stage 1 pressure ulcers
Stage 1: Intact skin with non-blanchable redness of a localized area usually over a bony prominence. Darkly pigmented skin may not have a visible blanching; in dark skin tones only it may appear with persistent blue or purple hues

B. Stage 2: Partial thickness loss of dermis presenting as a shallow open ulcer with a red or pink wound bed, without slough. May also present as an intact or open/ruptured blister

Enter Number [ ]
1. Number of Stage 2 pressure ulcers - If 0 → Skip to M0300C, Stage 3

Enter Number [ ]
2. Number of these Stage 2 pressure ulcers that were present upon admission/entry or reentry - enter how many were noted at the time of admission/entry or reentry

3. Date of oldest Stage 2 pressure ulcer - Enter dashes if date is unknown:

[ ][ ] – [ ][ ] – [ ][ ][ ][ ]
Month   Day   Year

C. Stage 3: Full thickness tissue loss. Subcutaneous fat may be visible but bone, tendon or muscle is not exposed. Slough may be present but does not obscure the depth of tissue loss. May include undermining and tunneling

Enter Number [ ]
1. Number of Stage 3 pressure ulcers - If 0 → Skip to M0300D, Stage 4

Enter Number [ ]
2. Number of these Stage 3 pressure ulcers that were present upon admission/entry or reentry - enter how many were noted at the time of admission/entry or reentry

D. Stage 4: Full thickness tissue loss with exposed bone, tendon or muscle. Slough or eschar may be present on some parts of the wound bed. Often includes undermining and tunneling

Enter Number [ ]
1. Number of Stage 4 pressure ulcers - If 0 → Skip to M0300E, Unstageable: Non-removable dressing

Enter Number [ ]
2. Number of these Stage 4 pressure ulcers that were present upon admission/entry or reentry - enter how many were noted at the time of admission/entry or reentry

---

M0300 continued on next page

Section M	Skin Conditions

M0300. Current Number of Unhealed (non-epithelialized) **Pressure Ulcers at Each Stage** - Continued

Enter Number ☐ Enter Number ☐	**E. Unstageable - Non-removable dressing:** Known but not stageable due to non-removable dressing/device 1. **Number of unstageable pressure ulcers due to non-removable dressing/device** - If 0 → Skip to M0300F, Unstageable: Slough and/or eschar 2. **Number of these unstageable pressure ulcers that were present upon admission/entry or reentry** - enter how many were noted at the time of admission/entry or reentry
Enter Number ☐ Enter Number ☐	**F. Unstageable - Slough and/or eschar:** Known but not stageable due to coverage of wound bed by slough and/or eschar 1. **Number of unstageable pressure ulcers due to coverage of wound bed by slough and/or eschar** - If 0 → Skip to M0300G, Unstageable: Deep tissue 2. **Number of these unstageable pressure ulcers that were present upon admission/entry or reentry** - enter how many were noted at the time of admission/entry or reentry
Enter Number ☐ Enter Number ☐	**G. Unstageable - Deep tissue:** Suspected deep tissue injury in evolution 1. **Number of unstageable pressure ulcers with suspected deep tissue injury in evolution** - If 0 → Skip to M0610, Dimension of Unhealed Stage 3 or 4 Pressure Ulcers or Eschar 2. **Number of these unstageable pressure ulcers that were present upon admission/entry or reentry** - enter how many were noted at the time of admission/entry or reentry

M0610. Dimensions of Unhealed Stage 3 or 4 Pressure Ulcers or Eschar
Complete only if M0300C1, M0300D1 or M0300F1 is greater than 0

If the resident has one or more unhealed (non-epithelialized) Stage 3 or 4 pressure ulcers or an unstageable pressure ulcer due to slough or eschar, identify the pressure ulcer with the largest surface area (length x width) and record in centimeters:

☐☐.☐ cm	**A. Pressure ulcer length:** Longest length from head to toe
☐☐.☐ cm	**B. Pressure ulcer width:** Widest width of the same pressure ulcer, side-to-side perpendicular (90-degree angle) to length
☐☐.☐ cm	**C. Pressure ulcer depth:** Depth of the same pressure ulcer from the visible surface to the deepest area (if depth is unknown, enter a dash in each box)

M0700. Most Severe Tissue Type for Any Pressure Ulcer

Enter Code ☐	Select the best description of the most severe type of tissue present in any pressure ulcer bed 1. **Epithelial tissue** - new skin growing in superficial ulcer. It can be light pink and shiny, even in persons with darkly pigmented skin 2. **Granulation tissue** - pink or red tissue with shiny, moist, granular appearance 3. **Slough** - yellow or white tissue that adheres to the ulcer bed in strings or thick clumps, or is mucinous 4. **Necrotic tissue (Eschar)** - black, brown, or tan tissue that adheres firmly to the wound bed or ulcer edges, may be softer or harder than surrounding skin 9. **None of the Above**

M0800. Worsening in Pressure Ulcer Status Since Prior Assessment (OBRA or Scheduled PPS) or Last Admission/Entry or Reentry
Complete only if A0310E = 0

Indicate the number of current pressure ulcers that were **not present or were at a lesser stage** on prior assessment (OBRA or scheduled PPS) or last entry. If no current pressure ulcer at a given stage, enter 0.

Enter Number ☐	**A. Stage 2**
Enter Number ☐	**B. Stage 3**
Enter Number ☐	**C. Stage 4**

Section M	Skin Conditions

M0900. Healed Pressure Ulcers
Complete only if A0310E = 0

Enter Code ☐	**A. Were pressure ulcers present on the prior assessment (OBRA or scheduled PPS)?** 0. **No** → Skip to M1030, Number of Venous and Arterial Ulcers 1. **Yes** → Continue to M0900B, Stage 2
	Indicate the number of pressure ulcers that were noted on the prior assessment (OBRA or scheduled PPS) that have completely closed (resurfaced with epithelium). If no healed pressure ulcer at a given stage since the prior assessment (OBRA or scheduled PPS), enter 0.
Enter Number ☐	**B. Stage 2**
Enter Number ☐	**C. Stage 3**
Enter Number ☐	**D. Stage 4**

M1030. Number of Venous and Arterial Ulcers

Enter Number ☐	**Enter the total number of venous and arterial ulcers present**

M1040. Other Ulcers, Wounds and Skin Problems

↓ Check all that apply

	Foot Problems
☐	**A. Infection of the foot** (e.g., cellulitis, purulent drainage)
☐	**B. Diabetic foot ulcer(s)**
☐	**C. Other open lesion(s) on the foot**
	Other Problems
☐	**D. Open lesion(s) other than ulcers, rashes, cuts** (e.g., cancer lesion)
☐	**E. Surgical wound(s)**
☐	**F. Burn(s)** (second or third degree)
☐	**G. Skin tear(s)**
☐	**H. Moisture Associated Skin Damage (MASD)** (i.e. incontinence (IAD), perspiration, drainage)
	None of the Above
☐	**Z. None of the above** were present

M1200. Skin and Ulcer Treatments

↓ Check all that apply

☐	**A. Pressure reducing device for chair**
☐	**B. Pressure reducing device for bed**
☐	**C. Turning/repositioning program**
☐	**D. Nutrition or hydration intervention** to manage skin problems
☐	**E. Pressure ulcer care**
☐	**F. Surgical wound care**
☐	**G. Application of nonsurgical dressings** (with or without topical medications) other than to feet
☐	**H. Applications of ointments/medications** other than to feet
☐	**I. Application of dressings to feet** (with or without topical medications)
☐	**Z. None of the above** were provided

Section N	Medications

N0300. Injections

Enter Days ☐	Record the number of days that injections of any type were received during the last 7 days or since admission/entry or reentry if less than 7 days. If 0 → Skip to N0410, Medications Received

N0350. Insulin

Enter Days ☐	A. Insulin injections - Record the number of days that insulin injections were received during the last 7 days or since admission/entry or reentry if less than 7 days
Enter Days ☐	B. Orders for insulin - Record the number of days the physician (or authorized assistant or practitioner) changed the resident's insulin orders during the last 7 days or since admission/entry or reentry if less than 7 days

N0410. Medications Received

Indicate the number of DAYS the resident received the following medications during the last 7 days or since admission/entry or reentry if less than 7 days. Enter "0" if medication was not received by the resident during the last 7 days

Enter Days ☐	A. Antipsychotic
Enter Days ☐	B. Antianxiety
Enter Days ☐	C. Antidepressant
Enter Days ☐	D. Hypnotic
Enter Days ☐	E. Anticoagulant (warfarin, heparin, or low-molecular weight heparin)
Enter Days ☐	F. Antibiotic
Enter Days ☐	G. Diuretic

Resident _____ Identifier _____ Date _____

Section O — Special Treatments, Procedures, and Programs

O0100. Special Treatments, Procedures, and Programs

Check all of the following treatments, procedures, and programs that were performed during the last **14 days**

	1. While NOT a Resident	2. While a Resident
1. While NOT a Resident — Performed *while NOT a resident* of this facility and within the *last 14 days*. Only check column 1 if resident entered (admission or reentry) IN THE LAST 14 DAYS. If resident last entered 14 or more days ago, leave column 1 blank. **2. While a Resident** — Performed *while a resident* of this facility and within the *last 14 days*	↓ Check all that apply ↓	
Cancer Treatments		
A. Chemotherapy	☐	☐
B. Radiation	☐	☐
Respiratory Treatments		
C. Oxygen therapy	☐	☐
D. Suctioning	☐	☐
E. Tracheostomy care	☐	☐
F. Ventilator or respirator	☐	☐
G. BiPAP/CPAP	☐	☐
Other		
H. IV medications	☐	☐
I. Transfusions	☐	☐
J. Dialysis	☐	☐
K. Hospice care	☐	☐
L. Respite care		☐
M. Isolation or quarantine for active infectious disease (does not include standard body/fluid precautions)	☐	☐
None of the Above		
Z. None of the above	☐	☐

O0250. Influenza Vaccine - Refer to current version of RAI manual for current flu season and reporting period

Enter Code ☐ **A.** Did the **resident receive the Influenza vaccine in this facility** for this year's Influenza season?
- 0. **No** → Skip to O0250C, If Influenza vaccine not received, state reason
- 1. **Yes** → Continue to O0250B, Date vaccine received

B. Date vaccine received → Complete date and skip to O0300A, Is the resident's Pneumococcal vaccination up to date?

☐☐ - ☐☐ - ☐☐☐☐
Month — Day — Year

Enter Code ☐ **C.** If Influenza vaccine not received, state reason:
- 1. **Resident not in facility** during this year's flu season
- 2. **Received outside of this facility**
- 3. **Not eligible** - medical contraindication
- 4. **Offered and declined**
- 5. **Not offered**
- 6. **Inability to obtain vaccine** due to a declared shortage
- 9. **None of the above**

O0300. Pneumococcal Vaccine

Enter Code ☐ **A.** Is the resident's Pneumococcal vaccination up to date?
- 0. **No** → Continue to O0300B, If Pneumococcal vaccine not received, state reason
- 1. **Yes** → Skip to O0400, Therapies

Enter Code ☐ **B.** If Pneumococcal vaccine not received, state reason:
- 1. **Not eligible** - medical contraindication
- 2. **Offered and declined**
- 3. **Not offered**

MDS 3.0 Nursing Home Comprehensive (NC) Version 1.10.3 Effective 04/01/2012   Page 29 of 40

Section O	Special Treatments, Procedures, and Programs

O0400. Therapies

A. Speech-Language Pathology and Audiology Services

Enter Number of Minutes
☐☐☐☐

1. **Individual minutes** - record the total number of minutes this therapy was administered to the resident **individually** in the last 7 days

Enter Number of Minutes
☐☐☐☐

2. **Concurrent minutes** - record the total number of minutes this therapy was administered to the resident **concurrently with one other resident** in the last 7 days

Enter Number of Minutes
☐☐☐☐

3. **Group minutes** - record the total number of minutes this therapy was administered to the resident as **part of a group of residents** in the last 7 days

If the sum of individual, concurrent, and group minutes is zero, ➝ skip to O0400A5, Therapy start date

Enter Number of Days
☐

4. **Days** - record the **number of days** this therapy was administered for **at least 15 minutes** a day in the last 7 days

5. **Therapy start date** - record the date the most recent therapy regimen (since the most recent entry) started

6. **Therapy end date** - record the date the most recent therapy regimen (since the most recent entry) ended - enter dashes if therapy is ongoing

☐☐ – ☐☐ – ☐☐☐☐
Month   Day   Year

☐☐ – ☐☐ – ☐☐☐☐
Month   Day   Year

B. Occupational Therapy

Enter Number of Minutes
☐☐☐☐

1. **Individual minutes** - record the total number of minutes this therapy was administered to the resident **individually** in the last 7 days

Enter Number of Minutes
☐☐☐☐

2. **Concurrent minutes** - record the total number of minutes this therapy was administered to the resident **concurrently with one other resident** in the last 7 days

Enter Number of Minutes
☐☐☐☐

3. **Group minutes** - record the total number of minutes this therapy was administered to the resident as **part of a group of residents** in the last 7 days

If the sum of individual, concurrent, and group minutes is zero, ➝ skip to O0400B5, Therapy start date

Enter Number of Days
☐

4. **Days** - record the **number of days** this therapy was administered for **at least 15 minutes** a day in the last 7 days

5. **Therapy start date** - record the date the most recent therapy regimen (since the most recent entry) started

6. **Therapy end date** - record the date the most recent therapy regimen (since the most recent entry) ended - enter dashes if therapy is ongoing

☐☐ – ☐☐ – ☐☐☐☐
Month   Day   Year

☐☐ – ☐☐ – ☐☐☐☐
Month   Day   Year

C. Physical Therapy

Enter Number of Minutes
☐☐☐☐

1. **Individual minutes** - record the total number of minutes this therapy was administered to the resident **individually** in the last 7 days

Enter Number of Minutes
☐☐☐☐

2. **Concurrent minutes** - record the total number of minutes this therapy was administered to the resident **concurrently with one other resident** in the last 7 days

Enter Number of Minutes
☐☐☐☐

3. **Group minutes** - record the total number of minutes this therapy was administered to the resident as **part of a group of residents** in the last 7 days

If the sum of individual, concurrent, and group minutes is zero, ➝ skip to O0400C5, Therapy start date

Enter Number of Days
☐

4. **Days** - record the **number of days** this therapy was administered for **at least 15 minutes** a day in the last 7 days

5. **Therapy start date** - record the date the most recent therapy regimen (since the most recent entry) started

6. **Therapy end date** - record the date the most recent therapy regimen (since the most recent entry) ended - enter dashes if therapy is ongoing

☐☐ – ☐☐ – ☐☐☐☐
Month   Day   Year

☐☐ – ☐☐ – ☐☐☐☐
Month   Day   Year

O0400 continued on next page

For Activity Programs   **187**

Section O	Special Treatments, Procedures, and Programs

O0400. Therapies - Continued

D. Respiratory Therapy

Enter Number of Minutes

[ ][ ][ ][ ]

Enter Number of Days

[ ]

1. **Total minutes** - record the total number of minutes this therapy was administered to the resident in the last 7 days
   If zero, → skip to O0400E, Psychological Therapy

2. **Days** - record the **number of days** this therapy was administered for **at least 15 minutes** a day in the last 7 days

E. Psychological Therapy (by any licensed mental health professional)

Enter Number of Minutes

[ ][ ][ ][ ]

Enter Number of Days

[ ]

1. **Total minutes** - record the total number of minutes this therapy was administered to the resident in the last 7 days
   If zero, → skip to O0400F, Recreational Therapy

2. **Days** - record the **number of days** this therapy was administered for **at least 15 minutes** a day in the last 7 days

F. Recreational Therapy (includes recreational and music therapy)

Enter Number of Minutes

[ ][ ][ ][ ]

Enter Number of Days

[ ]

1. **Total minutes** - record the total number of minutes this therapy was administered to the resident in the last 7 days
   If zero, → skip to O0450, Resumption of Therapy

2. **Days** - record the **number of days** this therapy was administered for **at least 15 minutes** a day in the last 7 days

O0450. Resumption of Therapy - Complete only if A0310C = 2 or 3 and A0310F = 99

Enter Code

[ ]

A. **Has a previous rehabilitation therapy regimen (speech, occupational, and/or physical therapy) ended, as reported on this End of Therapy OMRA, and has this regimen now resumed at exactly the same level for each discipline?**
   0. **No** → Skip to O0500, Restorative Nursing Programs
   1. **Yes**

B. **Date on which therapy regimen resumed:**

[ ][ ] – [ ][ ] – [ ][ ][ ][ ]
Month   Day   Year

O0500. Restorative Nursing Programs

Record the **number of days** each of the following restorative programs was performed (for at least 15 minutes a day) in the last 7 calendar days (enter 0 if none or less than 15 minutes daily)

Number of Days	Technique
[ ]	A. **Range of motion (passive)**
[ ]	B. **Range of motion (active)**
[ ]	C. **Splint or brace assistance**

Number of Days	Training and Skill Practice in:
[ ]	D. **Bed mobility**
[ ]	E. **Transfer**
[ ]	F. **Walking**
[ ]	G. **Dressing and/or grooming**
[ ]	H. **Eating and/or swallowing**
[ ]	I. **Amputation/prostheses care**
[ ]	J. **Communication**

MDS 3.0 Nursing Home Comprehensive (NC) Version 1.10.3 Effective 04/01/2012

Page 31 of 40

Section O	Special Treatments, Procedures, and Programs

O0600. Physician Examinations

Enter Days
[ ][ ] Over the last 14 days, **on how many days did the physician (or authorized assistant or practitioner) examine the resident?**

O0700. Physician Orders

Enter Days
[ ][ ] Over the last 14 days, **on how many days did the physician (or authorized assistant or practitioner) change the resident's orders?**

Section P	Restraints

P0100. Physical Restraints

Physical restraints are any manual method or physical or mechanical device, material or equipment attached or adjacent to the resident's body that the individual cannot remove easily which restricts freedom of movement or normal access to one's body

↓ **Enter Codes in Boxes**

Coding:		
		Used in Bed
	[ ]	A. Bed rail
	[ ]	B. Trunk restraint
	[ ]	C. Limb restraint
0. **Not used**	[ ]	D. Other
1. **Used less than daily**		**Used in Chair or Out of Bed**
2. **Used daily**	[ ]	E. Trunk restraint
	[ ]	F. Limb restraint
	[ ]	G. Chair prevents rising
	[ ]	H. Other

Section Q	Participation in Assessment and Goal Setting

Q0100. Participation in Assessment

Enter Code ☐
A. Resident participated in assessment
  0. No
  1. Yes

Enter Code ☐
B. Family or significant other participated in assessment
  0. No
  1. Yes
  9. No family or significant other available

Enter Code ☐
C. Guardian or legally authorized representative participated in assessment
  0. No
  1. Yes
  9. No guardian or legally authorized representative available

Q0300. Resident's Overall Expectation
Complete only if A0310E = 1

Enter Code ☐
A. Select one for resident's overall goal established during assessment process
  1. Expects to be **discharged to the community**
  2. Expects to **remain in this facility**
  3. Expects to be **discharged to another facility/institution**
  9. **Unknown or uncertain**

Enter Code ☐
B. Indicate information source for Q0300A
  1. **Resident**
  2. If not resident, then **family or significant other**
  3. If not resident, family, or significant other, then **guardian or legally authorized representative**
  9. **Unknown or uncertain**

Q0400. Discharge Plan

Enter Code ☐
A. Is active discharge planning already occurring for the resident to return to the community?
  0. No
  1. Yes → Skip to Q0600, Referral

Q0490. Resident's Preference to Avoid Being Asked Question Q0500B
Complete only if A0310A = 02, 06, or 99

Enter Code ☐
Does the resident's clinical record document a request that this question be asked only on comprehensive assessments?
  0. No
  1. Yes → Skip to Q0600, Referral
  8. Information not available

Q0500. Return to Community

Enter Code ☐
B. Ask the resident (or family or significant other if resident is unable to respond): **"Do you want to talk to someone about the possibility of leaving this facility and returning to live and receive services in the community?"**
  0. No
  1. Yes
  9. Unknown or uncertain

Q0550. Resident's Preference to Avoid Being Asked Question Q0500B Again

Enter Code ☐
A. Does the resident (or family or significant other or guardian, if resident is unable to respond) **want to be asked about returning to the community on all assessments?** (Rather than only on comprehensive assessments.)
  0. **No** - then document in resident's clinical record and ask again only on the next comprehensive assessment
  1. Yes
  8. Information not available

Enter Code ☐
B. Indicate information source for Q0550A
  1. **Resident**
  2. If not resident, then **family or significant other**
  3. If not resident, family or significant other, then **guardian or legally authorized representative**
  8. No information source available

Q0600. Referral

Enter Code ☐
Has a referral been made to the Local Contact Agency? (Document reasons in resident's clinical record)
  0. **No** - referral not needed
  1. **No** - referral is or may be needed (For more information see Section Q Care Area Assessment #20)
  2. **Yes** - referral made

Resident _____ Identifier _____ Date _____

Section V	Care Area Assessment (CAA) Summary

V0100. Items From the Most Recent Prior OBRA or Scheduled PPS Assessment
Complete only if A0310E = 0 and if the following is true for the **prior assessment**: A0310A = 01- 06 or A0310B = 01- 06

Enter Code
☐☐
A. Prior Assessment Federal OBRA Reason for Assessment (A0310A value from prior assessment)
01. **Admission** assessment (required by day 14)
02. **Quarterly** review assessment
03. **Annual** assessment
04. **Significant change in status** assessment
05. **Significant correction** to **prior comprehensive** assessment
06. **Significant correction** to **prior quarterly** assessment
99. None of the above

Enter Code
☐☐
B. Prior Assessment PPS Reason for Assessment (A0310B value from prior assessment)
01. **5-day** scheduled assessment
02. **14-day** scheduled assessment
03. **30-day** scheduled assessment
04. **60-day** scheduled assessment
05. **90-day** scheduled assessment
06. **Readmission/return** assessment
07. **Unscheduled assessment used for PPS** (OMRA, significant or clinical change, or significant correction assessment)
99. None of the above

C. Prior Assessment Reference Date (A2300 value from prior assessment)

☐☐ – ☐☐ – ☐☐☐☐
Month   Day   Year

Enter Score
☐☐
D. Prior Assessment Brief Interview for Mental Status (BIMS) Summary Score (C0500 value from prior assessment)

Enter Score
☐☐
E. Prior Assessment Resident Mood Interview (PHQ-9©) Total Severity Score (D0300 value from prior assessment)

Enter Score
☐☐
F. Prior Assessment Staff Assessment of Resident Mood (PHQ-9-OV) Total Severity Score (D0600 value from prior assessment)

For Activity Programs   **191**

Section V	Care Area Assessment (CAA) Summary

V0200. CAAs and Care Planning

1. Check column A if Care Area is triggered.
2. For each triggered Care Area, indicate whether a new care plan, care plan revision, or continuation of current care plan is necessary to address the problem(s) identified in your assessment of the care area. The Addressed in Care Plan column must be completed within 7 days of completing the RAI (MDS and CAA(s)). Check column B if the triggered care area is addressed in the care plan.
3. Indicate in the Location and Date of CAA Information column where information related to the CAA can be found. CAA documentation should include information on the complicating factors, risks, and any referrals for this resident for this care area.

A. CAA Results

Care Area	A. Care Area Triggered	B. Care Planning Decision	Location and Date of CAA Assessment documentation
	↓ Check all that apply ↓		
01. Delirium	☐	☐	
02. Cognitive Loss/Dementia	☐	☐	
03. Visual Function	☐	☐	
04. Communication	☐	☐	
05. ADL Functional/Rehabilitation Potential	☐	☐	
06. Urinary Incontinence and Indwelling Catheter	☐	☐	
07. Psychosocial Well-Being	☐	☐	
08. Mood State	☐	☐	
09. Behavioral Symptoms	☐	☐	
10. Activities	☐	☐	
11. Falls	☐	☐	
12. Nutritional Status	☐	☐	
13. Feeding Tube	☐	☐	
14. Dehydration/Fluid Maintenance	☐	☐	
15. Dental Care	☐	☐	
16. Pressure Ulcer	☐	☐	
17. Psychotropic Drug Use	☐	☐	
18. Physical Restraints	☐	☐	
19. Pain	☐	☐	
20. Return to Community Referral	☐	☐	

B. Signature of RN Coordinator for CAA Process and Date Signed

1. Signature

2. Date

☐☐ – ☐☐ – ☐☐☐☐
Month   Day   Year

C. Signature of Person Completing Care Plan Decision and Date Signed

1. Signature

2. Date

☐☐ – ☐☐ – ☐☐☐☐
Month   Day   Year

Section X	**Correction Request**

Identification of Record to be Modified/Inactivated - The following items identify the existing assessment record that is in error. In this section, reproduce the information EXACTLY as it appeared on the existing erroneous record, even if the information is incorrect. This information is necessary to locate the existing record in the National MDS Database.

X0150. Type of Provider

Enter Code ☐

Type of provider
1. **Nursing home (SNF/NF)**
2. **Swing Bed**

X0200. Name of Resident on existing record to be modified/inactivated

A. First name:

☐☐☐☐☐☐☐☐☐☐☐☐

C. Last name:

☐☐☐☐☐☐☐☐☐☐☐☐☐☐☐☐☐☐

X0300. Gender on existing record to be modified/inactivated

Enter Code ☐

1. **Male**
2. **Female**

X0400. Birth Date on existing record to be modified/inactivated

☐☐ – ☐☐ – ☐☐☐☐
Month   Day   Year

X0500. Social Security Number on existing record to be modified/inactivated

☐☐☐ – ☐☐ – ☐☐☐☐

X0600. Type of Assessment on existing record to be modified/inactivated

Enter Code ☐☐

A. **Federal OBRA Reason for Assessment**
   01. **Admission** assessment (required by day 14)
   02. **Quarterly** review assessment
   03. **Annual** assessment
   04. **Significant change in status** assessment
   05. **Significant correction** to prior **comprehensive** assessment
   06. **Significant correction** to prior **quarterly** assessment
   99. **None of the above**

Enter Code ☐☐

B. **PPS Assessment**
   PPS Scheduled Assessments for a Medicare Part A Stay
   01. **5-day** scheduled assessment
   02. **14-day** scheduled assessment
   03. **30-day** scheduled assessment
   04. **60-day** scheduled assessment
   05. **90-day** scheduled assessment
   06. **Readmission/return** assessment
   PPS Unscheduled Assessments for a Medicare Part A Stay
   07. **Unscheduled assessment used for PPS** (OMRA, significant or clinical change, or significant correction assessment)
   Not PPS Assessment
   99. **None of the above**

Enter Code ☐

C. **PPS Other Medicare Required Assessment - OMRA**
   0. **No**
   1. **Start of therapy** assessment
   2. **End of therapy** assessment
   3. **Both Start and End of therapy** assessment
   4. **Change of therapy** assessment

X0600 continued on next page

Section X	Correction Request

X0600. Type of Assessment - Continued

Enter Code	**D. Is this a Swing Bed clinical change assessment?** Complete only if X0150 = 2
⬚	0. **No**
	1. **Yes**

Enter Code	**F. Entry/discharge reporting**
⬚⬚	01. **Entry** tracking record
	10. **Discharge** assessment-**return not anticipated**
	11. **Discharge** assessment-**return anticipated**
	12. **Death in facility** tracking record
	99. **None of the above**

X0700. Date on existing record to be modified/inactivated - **Complete one only**

A. Assessment Reference Date - Complete only if X0600F = 99

⬚⬚ – ⬚⬚ – ⬚⬚⬚⬚
Month   Day   Year

B. Discharge Date - Complete only if X0600F = 10, 11, or 12

⬚⬚ – ⬚⬚ – ⬚⬚⬚⬚
Month   Day   Year

C. Entry Date - Complete only if X0600F = 01

⬚⬚ – ⬚⬚ – ⬚⬚⬚⬚
Month   Day   Year

Correction Attestation Section - Complete this section to explain and attest to the modification/inactivation request

X0800. Correction Number

Enter Number	
⬚⬚	**Enter the number of correction requests to modify/inactivate the existing record, including the present one**

X0900. Reasons for Modification - Complete only if Type of Record is to modify a record in error (A0050 = 2)

↓ **Check all that apply**

⬚	A. **Transcription error**
⬚	B. **Data entry error**
⬚	C. **Software product error**
⬚	D. **Item coding error**
⬚	E. **End of Therapy - Resumption (EOT-R) date**
⬚	Z. **Other error requiring modification** If "Other" checked, please specify: _____

X1050. Reasons for Inactivation - Complete only if Type of Record is to inactivate a record in error (A0050 = 3)

↓ **Check all that apply**

⬚	A. **Event did not occur**
⬚	Z. **Other error requiring inactivation** If "Other" checked, please specify: _____

Section X	Correction Request

X1100. RN Assessment Coordinator Attestation of Completion

A. Attesting individual's first name:

☐☐☐☐☐☐☐☐☐☐☐☐

B. Attesting individual's last name:

☐☐☐☐☐☐☐☐☐☐☐☐☐☐☐☐☐☐

C. Attesting individual's title:

D. Signature

E. Attestation date

☐☐ – ☐☐ – ☐☐☐☐
Month   Day   Year

Section Z — Assessment Administration

Z0100. Medicare Part A Billing

Enter Code	A. **Medicare Part A HIPPS code** (RUG group followed by assessment type indicator):
	[ ][ ][ ][ ][ ][ ][ ]
	B. **RUG version code:**
	[ ][ ][ ][ ][ ][ ][ ][ ][ ][ ]
Enter Code [ ]	C. **Is this a Medicare Short Stay assessment?** 0. **No** 1. **Yes**

Z0150. Medicare Part A Non-Therapy Billing

A. **Medicare Part A non-therapy HIPPS code** (RUG group followed by assessment type indicator):
[ ][ ][ ][ ][ ][ ][ ]
B. **RUG version code:**
[ ][ ][ ][ ][ ][ ][ ][ ][ ][ ]

Z0200. State Medicaid Billing (if required by the state)

A. **RUG Case Mix group:**
[ ][ ][ ][ ][ ][ ][ ][ ][ ]
B. **RUG version code:**
[ ][ ][ ][ ][ ][ ][ ][ ][ ]

Z0250. Alternate State Medicaid Billing (if required by the state)

A. **RUG Case Mix group:**
[ ][ ][ ][ ][ ][ ][ ][ ][ ]
B. **RUG version code:**
[ ][ ][ ][ ][ ][ ][ ][ ][ ]

Z0300. Insurance Billing

A. **RUG billing code:**
[ ][ ][ ][ ][ ][ ][ ][ ][ ]
B. **RUG billing version:**
[ ][ ][ ][ ][ ][ ][ ][ ][ ]

MDS 3.0 Nursing Home Comprehensive (NC) Version 1.10.3 Effective 04/01/2012   Page 39 of 40

Section Z — Assessment Administration

Z0400. Signature of Persons Completing the Assessment or Entry/Death Reporting

I certify that the accompanying information accurately reflects resident assessment information for this resident and that I collected or coordinated collection of this information on the dates specified. To the best of my knowledge, this information was collected in accordance with applicable Medicare and Medicaid requirements. I understand that this information is used as a basis for ensuring that residents receive appropriate and quality care, and as a basis for payment from federal funds. I further understand that payment of such federal funds and continued participation in the government-funded health care programs is conditioned on the accuracy and truthfulness of this information, and that I may be personally subject to or may subject my organization to substantial criminal, civil, and/or administrative penalties for submitting false information. I also certify that I am authorized to submit this information by this facility on its behalf.

Signature	Title	Sections	Date Section Completed
A.			
B.			
C.			
D.			
E.			
F.			
G.			
H.			
I.			
J.			
K.			
L.			

Z0500. Signature of RN Assessment Coordinator Verifying Assessment Completion

A. Signature: _____

B. Date RN Assessment Coordinator signed assessment as complete:

☐☐ – ☐☐ – ☐☐☐☐
Month — Day — Year

MDS 3.0 Nursing Home Comprehensive (NC) Version 1.10.3 Effective 04/01/2012   Page 40 of 40

Care Area Assessments (CAAs) are the system of deciding which types of interventions will be needed. They are worked by scoring the MDS and reviewing the results in the book *Resident Assessment System for Long-term Care*. By reviewing the CAAs, each health care professional will be able to determine if there is a specific treatment required for the resident. The treatment interventions triggered by using CAAs indicate the basic, minimum standard of treatment for residents in long-term care facilities. There are 20 identified CAAs:

- Delirium
- Cognitive Loss/Dementia
- Visual Function
- Communication
- ADL Functional/Rehab Potential
- Urinary Incontinence and Indwelling Catheter
- Psychosocial Well-Being
- Mood State
- Behavior Problem
- Activities
- Falls
- Nutritional Status
- Feeding Tubes
- Dehydration/Fluid Maintenance
- Dental Care
- Pressure Ulcers
- Psychoactive Drug Use
- Physical Restraints
- Pain
- Return to Community Referral

All professionals should be familiar with the MDS, the *Resident Assessment System for Long-term Care*, CAAs, and how to decide if a treatment intervention is indicated. *Chapter 12* provides an overview of many of the CAAs that may "trigger" the need for action by the professional. To help the reader develop a fuller understanding of the process, CAA examples have been included in this appendix. The CAAs in this book are from *Resident Assessment System for Long-term Care* published by the US Department of Commerce, National Technical Information Service.

The first four pages of forms show how the Activity CAA is worked for a man in, hopefully, a short-term stay while recovering from a fall. Following that are three Social Services CAAs: Psychosocial Well-Being, Mood State, and Behavioral Symptoms. The Social Services CAAs are based on the following case profile.

---

[1] This discussion of Care Area Assessments is taken from *Long Term Care for Activity Professionals, Social Services Professionals, and Recreational Therapists, 6th Edition* by Elizabeth (Betsy) Best-Martini, MS, CTRS, ACC, Mary Anne Weeks, MPH, SSC, Priscilla Wirth, MS, RHIA, published by Idyll Arbor. Used with permission.

Mrs. R has been living at home with her husband as caregiver. Up until the last few months he was able to handle her care himself. She recently began leaving the home unattended, has been calling 911 for being held as a "prisoner," and has begun to be combative with her husband. She was admitted to the hospital after being found 2 miles from home in her nightgown and barefoot. She was subsequently transferred to the nursing home after it was deemed that her husband could no longer provide for her care. Her history: secretary at a real estate office, very concerned with her appearance, very involved with community services and church.

10.   ACTIVITIES

Review of Indicators of Activities

	Activity preferences prior to admission (from interviews and record)	Supporting Documentation (Basis/reason for checking the item, including the location, date, and source (if applicable) of that information)
☑	• Passive	Describes himself as happy in his routine. Reading, TV, and radio are his main interests. Family involved in care. Resident interview 10/5/2010
☐	• Active	
☐	• Outside the home	
☑	• Inside the home	
☐	• Centered almost entirely on family activities	
☐	• Centered almost entirely on non-family activities	
☐	• Group (F0500E) activities	
☑	• Solitary activities	
☐	• Involved in community service, volunteer activities	
☐	• Athletic	
☑	• Non-athletic	

	Current activity pursuits (from interviews and record)	
☑	• Resident identifies leisure activities that interest this resident	States interest in any food-related events, especially coffee and donuts. Resident interview 10/5/2010
☑	• Self-directed or done with others and/or planned by others	
☐	• Activities resident pursues when visitors are present	
☑	• Scheduled programs in which resident participates	
☐	• Activities of interest not currently available or offered to the resident	

For Activity Programs

201

✓	Health issues that result in reduced activity participation	Supporting Documentation (Basis/reason for checking the item, including the location, date, and source (if applicable) of that information)
☑	• Indicators of depression or anxiety (D0200, D0500)	
☐	• Use of psychoactive medications (N0400A-D)	Recent peptic ulcer and edema with stiffness in legs. Resolving but still weak. Uses 3-pt walker. Needs wheelchair for long distance mobility.
☑	• Functional/mobility (G0110) or balance (G0300) problems; physical disability	
☐	• Cognitive deficits (C0500, C0700-C1000), including stamina, ability to express self (B0700), understand others (B0800), make decisions C1000)	
☑	• Unstable acute/chronic health problem (from record) (O0100)	Resident interview 10/5/2010
☐	• Chronic health conditions, such as incontinence (H0300, H0400) or pain (J0300)	
☐	• Embarrassment or unease due to presence of equipment, such as tubes, oxygen tank, or colostomy bag (H0100) (from observation, record)	H&P 10/5/2010
☐	• Receives numerous treatments(O0100) that limit available time/energy (from record)	PT Notes 10/5/2010
☑	• Performs tasks slowly due to reduced energy reserves (observation, record)	

✓	Environmental or staffing issues that hinder participation	
☐	• Physical barriers that prevent the resident from gaining access to the space where the activity is held (observation)	N/A
☐	• Need for additional staff responsible for social activities (observation)	
☐	• Lack of staff time to involve residents in current activity programs (observation)	
☐	• Resident's fragile nature results in feelings of intimidation by staff responsible for the activity (from observation, interviews, record)	

✓	Unique skills or knowledge the resident has that he or she could pass on to others (from interviews and record)	Supporting Documentation (Basis/reason for checking the item, including the location, date, and source (if applicable) of that information)
☐	• Games	N/A
☐	• Complex tasks such as knitting, or computer skills	
☐	• Topic that might interest others	

✓	Issues that result in reduced activity participation	
☐	• Resident is new to facility or has been in facility long enough to become bored with status quo (from interview, record)	Socialization was mainly at work, and with his wife and family.
☐	• Psychosocial well-being issues, such as shyness, initiative, and social involvement	
☐	• Socially inappropriate behavior (E0200)	Interacts with others but not
☐	• Indicators of psychosis (E0100A-C)	interested in making new
☐	• Feelings of being unwelcome, due to issues such as those already involved in an activity drawing boundaries that are difficult to cross (from observation, interview, record)	friends.
☐	• Limited opportunities for resident to get to know others through activities such as shared dining, afternoon refreshments, monthly birthday parties, reminiscence groups (from observation, facility activity calendar)	Wants to get out of his room and see "what is going on."
☐	• Available activities do not correspond to resident's values, attitudes, expectations (from interview, record)	Resident interview 10/5/2010
☑	• Long history of unease in joining with others (from interview, record)	

Input from resident and/or family/representative regarding the care area. (Questions/Comments/Concerns/Preferences/Suggestions)
Family wants to encourage him to walk to activities of interest to increase strength. Also suggest he be introduced to men with similar interests and history

Analysis of Findings		Care Plan Considerations
Review indicators and supporting documentation, and draw conclusions. Document: • Description of the problem; • Causes and contributing factors; and • Risk factors related to the care area.	Care Plan Y/N	Document reason(s) care plan will/ will not be developed.
Mobility limited due to resolving health condition. Although content with in-room activities, there is the risk of spending too much time alone. This risk could impact condition and mood as well as pressure sores.	Y	Care plan will focus on supporting therapy goals to increase ambulation through involvement in related activities.

Referral(s) to another discipline(s) is warranted (to whom and why): __No_____

Information regarding the CAA transferred to the CAA Summary (Section V of the MDS):
☑ Yes   ☐ No

7.   PSYCHOSOCIAL WELL-BEING

Review of Indicators of Psychosocial Well-Being

✓	Modifiable factors Relationship problems (from resident, family, staff interviews and clinical record)	Supporting Documentation (Basis/reason for checking the item, including the location, date, and source (if applicable) of that information)
☑	• Resident says or indicates he or she feels lonely — Recent decline in social involvement and associated loneliness can be sign of acute health complications and depression	Social interaction has declined with onset of dementia. Husband does not think she is aware of this.
☐	• Resident indicates he or she feels distressed because of decline in social activities	
☑	• Over the past few years, resident has experienced absence of daily exchanges with relatives and friends	Very involved with community service & church in the past.
☐	• Resident is uneasy dealing with others	
☑	• Resident has conflicts with family, friends, roommate, other residents, or staff	Recently combative with husband & difficult to redirect.
☐	• Resident appears preoccupied with the past and unwilling to respond to needs of the present	
☐	• Resident seems unable or reluctant to begin to establish a social role in the facility; may be grieving lost status or roles	H&P 10/25/2010 husband interview
☐	• Recent change in family situation or social network, such as death of a close family member or friend	

✓	Customary lifestyle (from resident, family, staff interviews and clinical record) (Section F)	
☑	• Was lifestyle more satisfactory to the resident prior to admission to the nursing home?	See above.
☑	• Are current psychosocial/relationship problems consistent with resident's long-standing lifestyle or is this relatively new for the resident?	Undetermined at this time if her loss of former lifestyle is evident to her.
☐	• Has facility care plan to date been as consistent as possible with resident's prior lifestyle, preferences, and routines (F0400, F0600, F0800)?	

✓	**Diseases and conditions** that may impede ability to interact with others	**Supporting Documentation** (Basis/reason for checking the item, including the location, date, and source (if applicable) of that information)
☐	• Delirium (C1600 = 1, Delirium CAA)	*Ongoing decline in recent year is the major contributory factor.*
☐	• Mental retardation (A1550)	
☐	• Alzheimer's disease (I4200)	
☐	• Aphasia (I4300)	
☑	• Other dementia (I4800)	
☐	• Depression (I5800)	

✓	**Health status factors** that may inhibit social involvement	
☑	• Decline in activities of daily living (G0110)	*Declines are due to above, unlikely to resolve. Social interactions are primarily inhibited by her inability to recognize family and staff.*
☐	• Health problem, such as falls (J1700, J1800), pain (J0300, J0800), fatigue, etc.	
☑	• Mood (D0200A1, D0300, D0500A1, D0600) or behavior (E0200) problem that impacts interpersonal relationships or that arises because of social isolation (See Mood State and Behavioral Symptoms CAAs)	
☑	• Change in communication (B0700, B0800), vision (B1000), hearing (B0200), cognition (C0100)	*family/staff interview 10/25/2010*
☑	• Medications with side effects that interfere with social interactions, such as incontinence, diarrhea, delirium, or sleepiness	

✓	**Environmental factors** that may inhibit social involvement	
☐	• Use of physical restraints (P0100)	*Not related to her reduced social interaction. See above.*
☑	• Change in residence leading to loss of autonomy and reduced self-esteem	
☐	• Change in room assignment or dining location or table mates	
☐	• Living situation limits informal social interaction, such as isolation precautions (O0100M)	

✓	Strengths to build upon (from resident, family, staff interviews and clinical record)	Supporting Documentation (Basis/reason for checking the item, including the location, date, and source (if applicable) of that information)
☐	• Activities in which resident appears especially at ease interacting with others	Was very proud of her accomplishments, took pride in her appearance. Very giving and concerned with others. Unsure if this can be built on with her decline in cognition and behavior. husband interview 11/25/2010
☐	• Certain situations appeal to resident more than others, such as small groups or 1:1 interactions rather than large groups	
☐	• Certain individuals who seem to bring out a more positive, optimistic side of the resident	
☑	• Positive traits that distinguished the resident as an individual prior to his or her illness	
☑	• What gave the resident a sense of satisfaction earlier in his or her life?	

For Activity Programs

207

Input from resident and/or family/representative regarding the care area.
(Questions/Comments/Concerns/Preferences/Suggestions)

Per husband: "Her appearance & behaviors just aren't who she was. I want her to be safe and cared for."

Analysis of Findings		Care Plan Considerations
Review indicators and supporting documentation, and draw conclusions. Document: • Description of the problem; • Causes and contributing factors; and • Risk factors related to the care area.	Care Plan Y/N	Document reason(s) care plan will/ will not be developed.
Mrs. R is no longer able to recognize her old friends or recall her previous lifestyle. She recognizes her husband but doesn't remember his visits. Not evident that she is distressed due to the above.	N	Decline in social involvement & conflicts with husband primarily due to her worsening dementia. No resolvable issues indentified. See Activity & Cognition CAA for intervention to maintain quality of life.

Referral(s) to another discipline(s) is warranted (to whom and why): __No__

Information regarding the CAA transferred to the CAA Summary (Section V of the MDS):
☑ Yes ☐ No

8. MOOD STATE

Review of Indicators of Mood

✓	Psychosocial changes	Supporting Documentation (Basis/reason for checking the item, including the location, date, and source (if applicable) of that information)
☑	• Personal loss	Per husband & staff not evident that she is aware of changes.
☑	• Recent move into or within the nursing home	
☐	• Recent change in relationships, such as illness or loss of a relative or friend	
☐	• Recent change in health perception, such as perception of being seriously ill or too ill to return home	H&P 11/20/2010 interviews 11/20/2010
☑	• Clinical or functional change that may affect the resident's dignity, such as new or worsening incontinence, communication, or decline	

✓	Clinical issues that can cause or contribute to a mood problem	
☐	• Relapse of an underlying mental health problem	Worsening dementia is the root cause of her poor appetite, restlessness, & poor concentration. Indicators present prior to admission & worsening per husband.
☐	• Psychiatric disorder (anxiety, depression, manic depression, schizophrenia, Post Traumatic Stress disorder (I5700 – I6100)	
☐	• Alzheimer's disease (I4200)	
☐	• Delirium (C1600)	
☐	• Delusions (E0100C)	
☐	• Hallucinations (E0100A)	
☑	• Communication problems (B0700, B0800)	
☑	• Decline in Activities of Daily Living (G0110 and clinical record)	interviews 11/20/2010 psych eval 10/30/2010
☐	• Infection (I1600 – I2500 and clinical record)	
☐	• Pain (J0300 or J0800)	
☐	• Cardiac disease (I0200 – I0900)	
☐	• Thyroid abnormality (I3400)	
☐	• Dehydration (J1550C and clinical record)	
☐	• Metabolic disorder (I2900 – I3400)	
☐	• Neurological disease (I4200 – I5500)	
☐	• Recent cerebrovascular accident (I4500)	
☑	• Dementia, cognitive decline (I4800 and clinical record)	
☐	• Cancer (I0100)	
☐	• Other	

For Activity Programs

✓	**Medications** (from medication administration record and preadmission records if new admission)	**Supporting Documentation** (Basis/reason for checking the item, including the location, date, and source (if applicable) of that information)
☐	• Antibiotics N0400F)	N/A
☐	• Anticholinergics	
☐	• Antihypertensives	
☐	• Anticonvulsants	
☐	• Antipsychotics (N0400A)	
☐	• Cardiac medications	
☐	• Cimetidine	
☐	• Clonidine	
☐	• Chemotherapeutic agents	
☐	• Digitalis	
☐	• Other	
☐	• Glaucoma medications	
☐	• Guanethidine	
☐	• Immuno-suppressive medications	
☐	• Methyldopa	
☐	• Narcotics	
☐	• Nitrates	
☐	• Propranolol	
☐	• Reserpine	
☐	• Steroids	
☐	• Stimulants	

✓	**Laboratory tests**	
☐	• Serum calcium	N/A
☐	• Thyroid function	
☐	• Blood glucose	
☐	• Potassium	
☐	• Porphyria	

Input from resident and/or family/representative regarding the care area.
(Questions/Comments/Concerns/Preferences/Suggestions)
Per husband: She has always been an upbeat person. I don't think she's depressed now. She doesn't seem unhappy, just confused.

Analysis of Findings		Care Plan Considerations
Review indicators and supporting documentation, and draw conclusions. Document: • Description of the problem; • Causes and contributing factors; and • Risk factors related to the care area.	Care Plan Y/N	Document reason(s) care plan will/ will not be developed.
Mood indicators of poor appetite, restlessness, and poor sleep. Lack of interest related to her worsening dementia	N	Indicators not related to mood decline but due to her dementia & resulting behaviors. See Behavior CAA.

Referral(s) to another discipline(s) is warranted (to whom and why): N

Information regarding the CAA transferred to the CAA Summary (Section V of the MDS):
☑ Yes   ☐ No

9. BEHAVIORAL SYMPTOMS

Review of Indicators of Behavioral Symptoms

✓	Seriousness of the behavioral symptoms (E0300, E0800, E0900, E1100)	Supporting Documentation (Basis/reason for checking the item, including the location, date, and source (if applicable) of that information)
☐	• Resident is immediate threat to self – IMMEDIATE INTERVENTION REQUIRED	Elopement/wandering no longer a danger in monitored environment.
☐	• Resident is immediate threat to others – IMMEDIATE INTERVENTION REQUIRED	

✓	Nature of the behavioral disturbance (resident interview, if possible; staff observations)	
☑	• ⟨Provoked or unprovoked⟩	Hx of wandering & being combative with redirection. No pattern to resistance to care. She is often very sweet & accepting. Responds well to face to face instruction.
☑	• Offensive or defensive	
☐	• Purposeful	
☐	• Occurs during specific activities, such as bath or transfers	
☑	• Pattern, such as certain times of the day, or varies over time	
☐	• Others in the vicinity or involved	
☐	• Reaction to a particular action, such as being physically moved	staff/husband interview 11/22/10
☑	• Resident appears to startle easily	H&P 11/10/10

Documentation in a SNAP

✓	Medication side effects that can cause behavioral symptoms (from medication records)	Supporting Documentation (Basis/reason for checking the item, including the location, date, and source (if applicable) of that information)
☑	• New medication	Medications readjusted with recent hospitalization to address escalation of behaviors. Good response & more manageable behaviors. No s/e noted. Not contributing
☑	• Change in dosage	
☐	• Antiparkinsonian drugs - may cause hypersexuality, socially inappropriate behavior	
☐	• Sedatives, centrally active antihypertensives, some cardiac drugs, anticholinergic agents can cause paranoid delusions, delirium	
☐	• Bronchodilators or other respiratory drugs, which can increase agitation and cause difficulty sleeping	H&P 11/10/10
☐	• Caffeine	
☐	• Nicotine	
☐	• Medications that impair impulse control, such as benzodiazepines, sedatives, alcohol (or any product containing alcohol, such as some cough medicine)	

✓	Illness or conditions that can cause behavior problems	
☐	• Long-standing mental health problem associated with the behavioral disturbances, such as schizophrenia, bipolar disorder, depression, anxiety disorder, post-traumatic stress disorder (I5700 – I6100)	No change in physical condition
☐	• New or acute physical health problem or flare-up of a known chronic condition	N/A
☐	• Delusions (E0100C)	H&P 11/10/10
☐	• Illusions (E0100B)	
☐	• Hallucinations (E0100A)	
☐	• Paranoia (from record)	
☐	• Constipation (H0600)	
☐	• Congestive heart failure (I0600)	
☐	• Infection (I1700 – I2500)	
☐	• Head injury (I5500 and clinical record)	
☐	• Diabetes (I2900)	
☐	• Pain (J0300, J0800)	
☐	• Fever (J1500A and record)	
☐	• Dehydration (J1550C and record; also see Dehydration CAA)	

✓	Factors that can cause or exacerbate the behavior (from observation, interview, record)	Supporting Documentation (Basis/reason for checking the item, including the location, date, and source (if applicable) of that information)
☐	• Frustration due to problem communicating discomfort or unmet need	*Startles if approached quickly but not an exaggerated response. Fear not expressed verbally or facially.*
☐	• Frustration, agitation due to need to urinate or have bowel movement	
☐	• Fear due to not recognizing caregiver	
☐	• Fear due to not recognizing the environment or misinterpreting the environment or actions of others	*per husband: her behaviors are improved from those at home*
☐	• Major unresolved sources of interpersonal conflict between the resident and family members, other residents, or staff (also see Psychosocial Well-Being CAA)	*per staff: seems ill at ease in large groups*
☑	• Recent change, such as new admission or a new unit, assignment of new care staff, or withdrawal from a treatment program	
☐	• Departure from normal routines	*interviews 11/20/10*
☐	• Sleep disturbance	
☑	• Noisy, crowded area	
☐	• Dimly lit area	
☐	• Sensory impairment, such as hearing or vision problem (B0200, B1000)	
☐	• Restraints (P0100)	
☐	• Fatigue	
☐	• Need for repositioning (M1200)	

✓	Cognitive status problems (also see Cognitive Loss CAT/CAA)	
☐	• Delirium (C1300) record (Delirium CAT)	*See previous notes. Dementia and cognition decline not reversible & and primary contributory factor to behaviors.*
☑	• Dementia (I4800)	
☐	• Recent cognitive loss (from record, interviews with family, etc.)	
☐	• Alzheimer's disease (I4200)	
☐	• Effects of cerebrovascular accident (I4500)	

✓	Other Considerations	Supporting Documentation (Basis/reason for checking the item, including the location, date, and source (if applicable) of that information)
☐	• May be communicating discomfort, personal needs, preferences, fears, feeling ill	
☐	• Persons exhibiting long-standing problem behaviors related to psychiatric conditions may place others in danger of physical assault, intimidation, or embarrassment and place themselves at increased risk of being stigmatized, isolated, abused, and neglected by loved ones or care givers	N/A
☐	• The actions and responses of family members and caregivers can aggravate or even cause behavioral outbursts	

Input from resident and/or family/representative regarding the care area.
(Questions/Comments/Concerns/Preferences/Suggestions)
She seems to be doing better here & with the medication changes. My goal is to have her safe and comfortable. I hope she remains able to walk and recognize me.

Analysis of Findings		Care Plan Considerations
Review indicators and supporting documentation, and draw conclusions. Document: • Description of the problem; • Causes and contributing factors; and • Risk factors related to the care area.	Care Plan Y/N	Document reason(s) care plan will/ will not be developed.
Decline in eating, ADL skills, sleeplessness, restlessness, cognition primarily due to unresolvable and worsening dementia. Risk factors include further cognitive decline, falls, incontinence, & decreased mobility.	Y	IDT will address risk factors & intervene to slow or minimize declines in areas itemized. IDT will seek pharmaceutical interventions to slow cognitive decline.

Referral(s) to another discipline(s) is warranted (to whom and why): PT/RTA to maintain amb & continence. MD for possible medication intervention. RD to avoid weight loss.

Information regarding the CAA transferred to the CAA Summary (Section V of the MDS):
☑ Yes   ☐ No

Appendix D.
Index to Regulations and References

RESOURCES

State Operations Manual (Pub 100-7) Appendix PP Centers for Medicare and Medicaid, Revision 70, 1-7-11. http://www.cms.gov/Manuals/IOM.

Long Term Care Facility Resident Assessment Instrument (RAI) User's Manual, MDS. 3.0, Centers for Medicare and Medicaid, Version V1.07 updated 9/20/2011. http://www.cms.gov/NursingHomeQualityInits/45_NHQIMDS30TrainingMaterials.asp The manual is listed in the Downloads section.

Nursing Home Compare (Website for consumer information and quality measures for facilities) Centers for Medicare and Medicaid. http://www.medicare.gov (search nursing home compare)

ABOUT THE AUTHOR

Ann G Uniack is a registered health information administrator. Although now retired, she has specialized in clinical record systems for skilled nursing facilities for more than forty-five years. Originally from Portland, Oregon, she received her Bachelor of Science in Medical Records Science from Seattle University.

Her professional activities have included election to Director of the California Health Information Association and President of the San Francisco Health Information Association. She has also served as a committee chair and member of various local, state, and national professional association committees. She has been honored by the California Health Information Association as their Distinguished Member in 1997 and received the Professional Achievement Award in 2007.

Articles written by Ann G Uniack have been regularly published in the CHIA Journal. She has been a speaker at many seminars on subjects such as documentation in the clinical record and ICD-9-CM coding.

www.ingramcontent.com/pod-product-compliance
Lightning Source LLC
Chambersburg PA
CBHW081811200326
41597CB00023B/4218